Hands Off!

70 Active Learning Strategies
for Exercise Science and Personal Training

Virginia S. Cowen, PhD

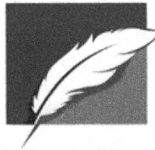

Pennate Press

ISBN 978-1-953891-32-7

Cataloging-in-Publication Data

Cowen, Virginia S., author
Hands Off! 70 active learning strategies for exercise science and personal training /
Virginia S. Cowen
ISBN 978-1-953891-32-7

Library of Congress Control Number: 2020920874

Product or corporate names which may be trademarked are included for informational purposes only with no intent to infringe.

First printing November 2020

Published by
Pennate Press
An imprint of IngeniousWellness
P.O. Box 83
Piermont, NY 10968

www.pennatepress.com

Preface

Peer practice instruction and lab activities can feel like a reward for students in exercise science, kinesiology, fitness instruction, and personal training. The perception of a hands on reward is for sitting through courses in science, psychology, and behavior. The difference is not entirely the content, but the instructional approaches used to cover material. Practice and labs are inherently active, didactic courses are sedentary and therefore more likely to be passive. When different instructional approaches are used it can be more difficult for students to integrate concepts.

Almost any topic can be crafted into a quality active learning experience that gets students on their feet, interacting, and doing something. Participation—even when it is not peer practice or a lab—helps students recall and apply concepts. These are essential steps in mastery of course material.

I heard a great deal of frustration from friends and colleagues forced into online teaching during the coronavirus pandemic. They had reverse-flipped their classrooms to use the synchronous distance learning for lectures and asking students to do activities as homework. The time spent with students was seated, looking at each other on a gallery of webcams without a lot of opportunity for interaction and engagement.

This book started out as a list of fun things that instructors could engage students when courses were taught in person or remotely. The original list grew into an outline, then paragraphs, then chapters. The result is a reference book that has been adapted for different areas of fitness and wellness. Regardless of whether an instructor is teaching in a degree program, certificate course, or continuing education activity, there are ideas in here for all formats for interaction and to help students master material.

Virginia S. Cowen, PhD

Contents

Introduction

Active learning is the purposeful engagement of students in the educational process. Instructional strategies that are experiential, experimental, or otherwise participatory provide students with the opportunities for engagement with material in a course. The self-practice and practice teaching in exercise science, kinesiology, and education for personal trainers and fitness instructors are hands on active learning. Hands off active learning offers another approach to teaching through participation, collaboration, and/or requiring students to seek information and find solutions.

Learning how to instruct clients, cue exercises, and use different types of fitness and testing equipment is only one part of training future professionals. . Basic science, psychology and movement science are foundational information upon which an effective exercise program is built. Critical thinking skills and the ability to integrate and apply information are essential. Active learning is a way to help students develop these skills and abilities.

Hands off active learning can easily be incorporated into Exercise science, kinesiology, and education for personal trainers and fitness instructors. Strategies can be used to help students review, apply, and integrate information. Grading and assessments can be built into active learning. Students learn from each other and about themselves which provides an informal assessment. Formative assessments can help students chart progress or identify needs for improvement. Reflection helps students recognize growth.

For instructors in exercise science, kinesiology, and education for personal trainers and fitness instructors programs that do not have formal education in teaching, fundamental information about teaching and learning is presented here for context. Knowledge progression and learning domains provide a framework for how students learn. Information about instructional design can be useful to guide selection of activities that meet educational standards and contact hour requirements.

Curriculum and Instruction

In education curriculum refers to content and instruction refers to how it is taught. Curriculum in exercise science, kinesiology, and education for personal trainers and fitness instructors includes exercises as well as foundational information from anatomy, physiology, movement science, ethics, and teaching strategies. Instruction in exercise science, kinesiology, and education for personal trainers and fitness instructors may include lecture, demonstration, self-practice, observation, and practice teaching. As students progress through a degree program, certification training, or a workshop it is expected that they will progress in their knowledge and be able to apply what they learn. Engaging instructional strategies can facilitate the path from student to future professional.

Knowledge Progression

Benjamin Bloom's Taxonomy of Educational Objectives is a well-known model that outlines the progression of learning in the cognitive domain. Knowledge, comprehension, application, analysis, synthesis, and evaluation are areas of learning that can also be viewed as a hierarchy for the complexity of course content. It is not enough for a student to be able to regurgitate information. Rather, students need to be able to recognize, recall, and utilize information by engaging with course material to explore issues or solve problems.

Activities used when material is introduced can help students become comfortable with terms, definitions, and concepts on a general level. More complex activities can be used to promote critical thinking when material is applied and integrated. For example, helping students identify when and how modify an exercise for a client. Building these ideas a session or the overall curriculum helps map the learning progression from the level at which information is introduced to where it is utilized. In order to effectively utilize information, students must be led through the progression of review, application, and integration. This can be accomplished with active learning strategies.

Learning Domains

Use of movement, role-play, discussion, reflection, research, and other participatory approaches are student-centered because they engage students in different domains of learning: cognitive, psychomotor, and affective.

The *cognitive* domain involves thinking. This goes beyond simple repetition of information to recognize different levels of learning and use of didactic information. Bloom's Taxonomy is often used to provide a framework for lesson plans, particularly learning objectives that increase in complexity from introduction through mastery of information: knowledge, comprehension, application, analysis, synthesis, evaluation.

The *psychomotor* domain is kinesthetic. It includes movement, motor skills, and coordination. The psychomotor domain also includes touch (the haptic sense) and the ability to sense by using touch (feeling.) Teaching and learning in the psychomotor domain fundamentally involves observation, imitation, and practice. On a more advanced level, the psychomotor domain also includes adaptation when the student makes adjustments to a skill or movement.

The *affective* domain involves feelings and perceptions. It includes interests, attitudes, and emotions expressed through receiving, responding to, and valuing information. This is the domain where professionalism comes into play.

While self-practice and practice teaching sessions emphasize the psychomotor domain, the requirements for teaching exercise and fitness are more substantial. Comprehensive learning includes integration of fundamentals and knowledge about the exercises with a professional demeanor from the intake interview, to assessment, the session, and through to follow up and reassessment. Recognizing opportunities for student engagement at all stages of this learning process can help to embrace different learning preferences while at the same time reinforcing course material.

Instructional Design

Successful active learning requires instructors and students to be engaged in the activity. It can be challenging to take fun activities seriously, so instructors need to set a tone and work to manage the classroom. Training students to take active learning seriously is essential for any activity to be a success, so selecting where and when to include active learning strategies requires careful consideration.

Students can work individually, in small groups, or as teams. Activities can involve movement, observation, collaborative activities, project-based activities, study skills, peer teaching, games, team-based learning, and/or case-based learning. As students get used to active learning formats, it can be very rewarding. There are different ways to incorporate active learning strategies in a class.

Flipped Classroom

For face-to-face or online synchronous courses, a flipped classroom can be used to engage students. A flipped classroom requires students to complete preparatory work prior to class, and then during class they apply, practice, or engage in creative activities. In order for this instructional strategy to be effective, students may need incentive to prepare for class.

Experiential learning, similar to a lab, provides an opportunity for an applied or kinesthetic experience. Movement and motion can be used to help students embody information from anatomy & physiology or movement science. Collaborative activities, role-play, and team-based learning can foster communication and leadership skills.

The flipped classroom is often already used for online asynchronous courses that require viewing recorded lectures prior to participation in discussion forums, but additional active learning strategies can be implemented to engage students in other ways. Creative projects, peer teaching, games, and even movement activities can make asynchronous classes more interactive.

Formative Assessment

Activities can be selected to provide students with the opportunity for informal assessments when instructors observe student participation. Self-assessment naturally occurs during activities when students recognize how well they know material and are able to apply concepts. Assignments that are products of active learning can also be used as assessments of student performance.

Because active learning requires students to show evidence that they know, can apply, or synthesize material, activities provide an opportunity for instructors to informally assess the class as a whole. Giving students the chance to ask questions, seek clarification, and use resource material can help them become more proactive and self-directed in their learning.

Review

Active learning strategies can provide an excellent format for review sessions. Often review sessions involve students asking questions that are answered by the instructor. Structuring activities so that they require review of material makes review more student focused. Collaborative activities, games, and peer teaching can cover a large amount of material. Case-based learning that poses complex problems also has potential to cover a large amount of material while requiring students to apply and integrate knowledge. Games, movement, or observational activities can help students recall and remember information through the combination of visual, verbal, auditory, and kinesthetic cues.

Planning

There is a misperception that active learning requires instructors to be creative. Organization and planning are more important than creativity. Pairing an activity with course material and a learning outcome does not require creativity, just lesson planning. A feedback loop can be used by asking students to identify individual learning objectives before the activity. Then at the end of the activity they can be invited to reflect on how well they met their own learning objectives. To select a suitable activity, begin with course content and learning objectives for a session. Necessary materials should be secured, class space laid out, and an adequate description of the activity prepared. Once students become familiar with certain types of activities, those can be repeated with different content.

Instructional Time

Active learning does not require more—or less—classroom time than conventional teaching methods. Strategizing and preparation can take time for instructors who are new to active learning or are teaching a course or workshop for the first time. Starting small can help instructors become skilled at managing a class. Leave adequate time at the beginning of class for pre-briefing. This should include directions, formation of groups, and defining roles. All details about materials students are expected to produce (i.e. summary, document, or presentation) should be included in the pre-briefing. As students get used to active learning sessions, the amount of time needed for pre-briefing will decrease.

Facilitation

Active learning sessions can seem chaotic, so facilitation is essential to keep students on-track and on-task. Regardless of whether students are working individually or in groups, instructors should observe, answer questions, give in-the-moment feedback, and (where applicable) recommend resources. Instructors should be accessible during the activity.

For face-to-face classes, being present in the room and moving around to observe creates informal opportunities for interaction without interruption of the activity. This is not the same in online classes. For synchronous online sessions being visible on camera, responding to questions posed verbally or using the chat feature does convey presence. But the opportunity for casual interaction and feeling instructor presence is diminished unless the instructor makes effort. Instructor presence in the asynchronous environment needs to be more purposeful since there is a lack of direct communication. Monitoring student attendance (i.e. log ins) and reviewing student participation is not easily sensed by students. Communicating with them during learning activities by contributing feedback, asking for clarifications, and making suggestions conveys a sense of presence. Because active learning aims to be student centered, the instructor should be visible but can be in the background.

Reflection and Debriefing

At the end of the active learning session, the instructor should bring the class together to draw the activity to a close. This should be brief, succinct, and reference the objectives of the activity to stress relevance to the course. The instructor can summarize the activity and review the objectives. Then a few individual students or a spokesperson for a few groups can share a reflection with the class. The instructor can summarize how the material covered fits into the overall course. If a feedback loop was used, students can be asked to write a brief self-assessment on how well they met their own objectives. Additional ideas are presented in the Appendix.

Evaluation

Evaluation of an activity is important to gain insight from students about the activity and how it contributed to learning. It can also help to identify aspects of the activity that could be enhanced or improved. Brief surveys can be completed immediately after the session. Students can also reflect in a group discussion to provide an informal evaluation.

How to use this Book

The core of this book is divided into chapters that include different types of active learning strategies: movement-based, observational, collaborative, project-based, study skills, peer teaching, games, team-based learning, case-based learning, and creative case scenarios. Within the chapters, each activity has a two-page summary. This includes a brief description of the activity along with details for execution. Materials needed and instructional approaches will differ for face-to-face and distance-learning formats. The appendix provides information and examples to help instructors with ideas for active learning implementation.

Some topic areas are better-suited to different types of activities. Most active learning strategies can be adapted to different stages of learning. Recognizing diverse needs of students is essential to create inclusive and culturally competent activities. A general summary is provided here, specifics are listed for each active learning strategy.

Materials and Implementation

A range of materials can be employed to facilitate active learning. For each activity, materials needed, implementation ideas, and modifications are listed. Some activities are not suited for all learning environments. A double dash ("--") is used to indicate an activity that cannot be modified or delivered in a particular format.

For **face-to-face** classes, whiteboard, sticky notes, and flip charts with markers can be used for whole-class activities or small groups. Blank paper, notecards, pens/pencils can be used for individual or group activities. Laptops, tablets, or smartphones (with internet access) can be used to search databases for reference material. Smartphones or tablets can be used to make videos.

For **online synchronous** or **online asynchronous** courses, the materials will be contingent upon what is available in the learning management system. This can include presentations, discussion forums, breakout rooms, whiteboards, wikis, quizzes, games, and different ways to share student-prepared documents, presentations, and/or videos.

Students in exercise science, kinesiology, and education for personal trainers and fitness instructors programs are always expected to wear clothing that permits safe movement. Exercise clothing is not necessarily required for course content that is not movement based (e.g. anatomy & physiology.) A note is included about clothing and footwear for instructional strategies that involve movement. For any remote instruction, students should also have space that is free of obstructions and is adequate to permit movement.

Topic Areas

Exercise science, kinesiology, and education for personal trainers and fitness instructors involves different topics and sometimes different courses depending upon the program. Students can enroll in courses on just mat, different apparatus, or special populations.

Specific content can vary, but there are general topic areas that can be used to categorize learning activities:

— Anatomy & physiology
— Movement science
— Assessment and evaluation
— Exercise program design
— Ethics

While it is easy to think of using a movement-based activity for movement science and a cognitive activity for assessment and evaluation, switching this around can substantially enhance learning. For example, *Silly Walks* is a movement activity that can be used to review motor disorders in assessment and evaluation. *Fuzzy or Clear* is a peer teaching strategy that could be used to review movement science concepts.

The laboratory component of traditional anatomy & physiology courses include a range of active learning instructional approaches for experiential learning. This includes observation of models, dissection, tissue testing, and other hands-on activities. Exercise science, kinesiology, and education for personal trainers and fitness instructors programs lack an anatomy laboratory, but a similar approach can be used by active learning strategies. *Simon Says*, *Dancers 1* and *Dolly and Me* are examples of strategies that can be used to help students review and apply anatomy & physiology concepts through experiential learning.

Professional ethics are an interesting topic in exercise science, kinesiology, and education for personal trainers and fitness instructors when some students have a clinical background and others do not. Role-play is an active learning strategy can be used to have students observe, model, or work through solutions to issues that might arise related to scope of practice. Other topics in ethics can be covered in *Dominos*, *Create a Study Guide*, and *I Could Teach That* to help students review and apply ideas.

The depth of material in exercise science, kinesiology, and education for personal trainers and fitness instructors provides an array of opportunities to get students involved and engaged with course material—beyond simply practicing teaching each other exercises. Active learning strategies can help students remember, analyze, and synthesize information from different areas in the curriculum. That can help them think more critically in exercise program design. As students learn to work in a self-directed manner, it can plant the seeds for lifelong learning.

Learning Stage Adaptation Examples

This book provides suggestions to adapt each active learning strategy to three different stages in the progression of learning: review, application, and integration. All activities are not suited to each stage. Examples of activities are provided to spark ideas and help instructors get started. However, this book is not intended to be prescriptive for each and every scenario. When an instructor identifies a gap or need at a specific learning stage, selection and implementation of an activity can help students bridge a knowledge gap.

Using active learning to help students **review** material can provide ways to recognize and utilize information that is more meaningful than simply trying to memorize and recall. *In a Flash* and *Got Your Back* are two games that use fun and creative approaches to go through terms and Definitions. *Clinic Role-Play* requires students to identify and extract essential information. *Explain that to Grandma* helps students define terms by requiring them to rephrase a complicated concept and avoid jargon.

Application of course material and concepts requires students to be able to make connections and solve problems. Activities can be structured to help students make sense of abstract ideas. For example, when students have difficulty with muscle anatomy, an activity like *Puppet Master* and *Fashion Models 2* can be used to connect origins and insertions with actions and movements. *Rowing Team* can be used to help students explore ways that different terms relate to each other. *Creative Case Studies* provides an opportunity to extract information from a source and use it to develop a cohesive scenario.

Integration occurs when students utilize material and concepts from different areas in a curriculum. Using active learning strategies can be helpful, especially when the activity involves a game. *Connect the Dots* can be used to organize anatomy & physiology terms. *Daisy Chain* can be structured to have students work through a complex disease or disorder. The game aspect of the activity can make the content seem less daunting.

It can be especially useful to use an activity to review material and then revisit it later in the curriculum with the goal of application or integration of material. *Calisthenics 1* is a movement-based activity that can be used for a review of joint movements. It can also be used with the goal of having students integrate joint movements with concepts from movement science. *Sports Stars 1* is another movement-based activity that can be used to promote understanding of movement science concepts. It can also be used to encourage strategies to support exercise program design.

Diversity Considerations

When choosing active learning strategies, the needs and abilities of the students must be taken into account. That means inclusiveness for physical disabilities, learning disabilities, and English-language learners. It also requires balancing needs of slower learners with overeager or overachieving students. Care in composing small groups can help to create balanced opportunities for all participants when slower learners are paired with higher-achieving students. This is especially important for peer learning and collaborative activities.

Students in exercise science, kinesiology, and education for personal trainers and fitness instructors, like other areas of post-secondary education, have different levels of academic preparedness. Using active learning for informal assessments provides opportunities for the instructor to gauge the extent to which students are mastering material and concepts. This is different than the student's ability to perform or cue an exercise. For students who struggle to learn, informal assessment is less risky than waiting for a high-stakes assessment like a final test out or certification examination. Students who need help can be identified earlier and directed to resources and strategies to help them succeed.

Depending upon the characteristics of the surrounding community, students may come from different cultures and socioeconomic backgrounds. Collectively, this means that students may have different expectations, knowledge, and attitudes. They can also have different communication styles, collaboration approaches, and willingness to speak up in class. Activities that allow students to leverage or highlight their own culture or background can contribute to cultural competence for the class as a whole. That may arm the students with knowledge and skills to better serve their community in the future.

Kinesthetic Activities

Strike a Pose

Have students take turns assuming a pose in front of the class to act as a model. The rest of class analyzes the position of the body using concepts from anatomy and movement science. For novice learners, this can be done with the instructor guiding the class to look at specific areas of the body (e.g. the shoulder or hip joint.) After students are comfortable with this activity, they can follow a sequence (e.g. from feet to head) to analyze the position.

This activity is good for quick reviews, to demonstrate rapid recall, and to encourage familiarity in using movement and anatomical terminology. It can also be used to practice assessing posture.

Materials and Implementation

Students should wear clothing and footwear that permits movement.

Face-to-Face

This activity works well in face-to-face classes.

Online Synchronous

Students can demonstrate poses for each other using a webcam.

Online Asynchronous

Students could take turns serving as a model by uploading a photo of themselves in a pose to a discussion forum for other students to analyze.

Topic Areas

Anatomy & physiology

Movement science

Assessment and evaluation

Learning Stage Adaptation Examples

Review

Identify where an area of the poser's body is in relation to the coronal, transverse, or sagittal plane.

Basic positions of joints (e.g. what is the position of the right elbow?)

Agonist muscles used to produce a joint position.

Antagonist muscles that are elongated to accommodate a joint position.

Review movement science concepts: base of support, center of gravity, types of levers.

Application

Complex joint positions with analysis agonist and antagonist muscles involved in relevant actions.

Identify a movement that could come before or after the pose to create a logical movement sequence.

Integration

List active or passive insufficiencies that might make it difficult for someone else to assume the same position.

Identify diseases or disorders that might make it difficult for someone else to assume the same position.

Diversity Considerations

Some students may not be comfortable being the center of attention, so they may be reluctant to serve as the poser.

Dance Break

Separate the class into two groups. One group dances while the other group observes. Play some fun dance music while the dancers keep dancing until the instructor stops the music. When the music stops, the dancers must freeze in position. The other group analyzes the position of their bodies using concepts from anatomy or movement science.

This can be a fun activity to help the students review, and a stress reliever when they get to dance and listen to music.

Materials and Implementation

Students should wear clothing and footwear that permits movement.

Face-to-Face

This activity works well in face-to-face classes.

Online Synchronous

This can be easily executed with students using webcams with a small group of students. To keep the discussion organized, the instructor might need to call on observers so that all students can participate.

Online Asynchronous

--

Topic Areas

Anatomy & physiology

Movement science

Assessment and evaluation

Learning Stage Adaptation Examples

Review

Identify where an area of the poser's body is in relation to the coronal, transverse, or sagittal plane.

Basic positions of joints (e.g. what is the position of the right elbow?)

Agonist muscles used to produce a joint position.

Antagonist muscles that are elongated to accommodate a joint position.

Review movement science concepts: base of support, center of gravity, types of levers.

Compare and contrast open-chain and closed-chain joint positions

Application

Complex joint positions with analysis agonist and antagonist muscles involved in relevant actions.

Identify a movement that could come before, or after the pose to create a logical movement sequence.

Integration

List active or passive insufficiencies that might make it difficult for someone else to assume the same position.

Identify diseases or disorders that might make it difficult for someone else to assume the same position.

Diversity Considerations

Some religious and spiritual groups prohibit dancing so students may not feel able to participate.

Using music from different genres and cultures can be interesting.

Simon Says

The playground game *Simon Says* can be useful to help students review muscles, joint movements, and movement science concepts. The instructor tells students to demonstrate a specific movement. Sometimes the instruction is prefaced with "Simon says..." and other times not. The students should only execute a movement when the phrase "Simon says" is used. If a student moves when the instructor does not say "Simon says," then that is considered incorrect.

This can be played like a knockout game. Any students who make the wrong movement or move when the instructor does not say "Simon says" are considered out of the game, and sit down. The other students keep the game going until one student is left.

Materials and Implementation

Students should wear clothing and footwear that permits movement.

Face-to-Face

This activity works well in face-to-face classes with all students participating.

Online Synchronous

This can be easily executed with students using webcams.

Online Asynchronous

--

Topic Areas

Anatomy & physiology

Movement science

Learning Stage Adaptation Examples

Review

Contract a specific muscle to produce a movement (e.g. Simon says: flex your right biceps brachii.)

Perform a funny movement (e.g. Simon says: flex your knees but not your hips)

Application

Demonstrate closed or open chain joint positions (e.g. Simon says: show me an open chain position of the left leg.)

Perform a movement that engages a muscle or muscle group in a certain way (e.g. Simon says: show me eccentric contraction of the quadriceps muscle group.)

Integration

Perform a complex movement (e.g. Simon says: Show me any combination of two movements in the sagittal plane that also involve a wide base of support)

Diversity Considerations

Struggling students may feel bad if they lose. They may become disinterested when they have to sit out. Using positive reinforcement can encourage these students.

Calisthenics 1

Calisthenics are repetitive movements using a person's own body weight to exercise. They are also movements that can be used to create a movement-based review. In this activity, students take turns demonstrating calisthenics while the remainder of the class analyzes movements.

Ask a student volunteer to start demonstrating a specific exercise at a comfortable pace. The instructor calls out one joint and the class needs to say the movements for that joint repeatedly in real time during the demonstration. The class can chant the movement to change the pace to have the demonstration speed up or slow down.

Materials and Implementation

The students who volunteer to demonstrate should wear clothing and footwear that permits movement.

An exercise mat is needed.

Face-to-Face

This activity works well in face-to-face classes.

Online Synchronous

This can be easily executed with students using webcams. To keep the activity organized, a single student could analyze while another performs calisthenics.

There should be adequate space to move comfortably and view students from the camera's position.

Online Asynchronous

--

Topic Areas

Anatomy & physiology

Movement science

Learning Stage Adaptation Examples

Review

Ask a student volunteer to perform jumping jacks or arm circles, then direct the class to describe movement at the shoulder in the sequence it occurs.

Application

After the class describes the movements, have them review and antagonist muscles involved in the movements (e.g. biceps brachii and triceps brachii in a push-up.)

Do this activity in a series. Ask the student volunteer to select a calisthenics exercise that is connected in some way to what the previous student did. After the movements have been described the class has to successfully guess the connection. (e.g. knees are flexed during a squat and an abdominal curl-up)

Integration

Ask the students to discuss or demonstrate a variation that would vary base of support (for standing exercises) or change the load on a joint/lever (for exercises that are seated or lying down)

Link a repetitive stress injury or injury pattern associated with this exercise to a potentially helpful exercise for a client to use for self-care at home.

Diversity Considerations

Students who are not physically fit may be reluctant to serve as the demonstrator or may have difficulty sustaining the exercise. Modifications to exercises can help accommodate that so everyone can take turns as the model at their own level of ability.

Calisthenics 2

In this version of the activity, all students exercise. This activity begins with the instructor calling out a calisthenics exercise. The whole class engages in the movement. While they are moving, the instructor calls out a joint. The students need to describe the action or position of that joint while they continue to perform the exercise.

Materials and Implementation

Students should wear clothing and footwear that permits movement.

Face-to-Face

This activity works well in face-to-face classes.

An exercise mat is needed.

Online Synchronous

This can be easily executed with students using webcams. Exercise mats are needed. There should be adequate space to move comfortably and view students from camera position.

Online Asynchronous

Students could be assigned an exercise that they film themselves demonstrating and describing. The videos can be uploaded to a folder for the class to compare and contrast in a written forum.

Topic Areas

Anatomy & physiology

Movement science

Learning Stage Adaptation Examples

Review

The class performs lunges while describing the movement of one joint before switching to another (e.g. focusing on the knee, the students say flexion every time they lunge and flex the knee.) For a face-to-face class they can walk in a circle moving clockwise around the classroom. For an online class, they can stand facing a webcam.

The class can perform regular partial curl-ups (e.g. extension of the vertebral column occurs in the lowering phase of the movement.)

Application

Introduce a variation to an exercise and have the students analyze how it changes. Examples:

— Short box with flat back vs. short box with twist
— Hundreds with a ball between the feet vs. behind the head

Integration

Have the students describe movement science concepts in addition to muscle and joint movements. Example: the difference in center of gravity that occurs when performing push up.

Diversity Considerations

Students who are not physically fit may be reluctant to participate or may have difficulty sustaining the exercise. Modifications to exercises can help accommodate that so everyone participates.

Calisthenics 3

Students take turns drawing cards from a deck. Each card has a specific joint movement. The students must select a repetitive calisthenics exercise that includes that joint movement. They perform their selection and keep going until the rest of the class successfully guesses what joint movement was on the card.

Materials and Implementation

Students should wear clothing and footwear that permits movement. An exercise mat is needed.

Face-to-Face

This activity works well in face-to-face classes.

Online Synchronous

This can be easily executed with students using webcams. To keep the discussion organized, the instructor might need to have a single student analyze while another performs calisthenics.

There should be adequate space to move comfortably and view students from the camera's position.

Online Asynchronous

Students could be assigned an exercise that they film themselves demonstrating and describing. The videos can be uploaded to a folder for the class to compare and contrast in a written forum.

Topic Areas

Anatomy & physiology

Movement science

Learning Stage Adaptation Examples

Review

The class should attempt to describe all joint movements while the student volunteer performs the exercise. Once they say the correct movement, another student takes a turn and selects a different card.

Application

After the students successfully identify the joint movement, they review agonist and antagonist muscles involved in that movement.

Integration

Have the students propose a variation that changes a movement science concept (e.g. widen feet in an exercise for a larger base of support.)

Diversity Considerations

Until students are comfortable in the class, some may be reluctant to think on their feet in front of everyone. Novice students could consult with the instructor after they think of an exercise to perform.

Students may have difficulty sustaining the exercise while the class tries to guess the movement. They should be encouraged to take breaks as needed.

Mime Time 1

This activity involves demonstration of everyday tasks using mimed movements. The instructor can prepare a deck of index cards with different everyday tasks. One at a time, students draw a card and then silently perform movements of that activity. They keep doing the mimed activity until the rest of the class successfully guesses what it is and then discuss the movements involved in performing that activity.

Materials and Implementation

Students should wear clothing and footwear that permits movement.

Face-to-Face

Prepared deck of index cards with a variety of everyday movements

This activity works well in face-to-face classes. It can also be funny if students get creative in how they mime.

Online Synchronous

This can be easily executed with students using webcams. The instructor would need to assign each student a task using chat so the other students cannot see what will be done.

There should be adequate space to move comfortably and view students from camera position.

Online Asynchronous

Students could prepare short videos of themselves. These could be shared to a discussion forum for other students in the class to analyze

Topic Areas

Anatomy & physiology

Movement science

Assessment and evaluation

Learning Stage Adaptation Examples

Review

Students are asked to describe basic movements that are being demonstrated and the joints/muscles involved. Examples: Walking up or down stairs, carrying groceries, stirring a pot on the stove, or putting on a sweater

Application

More complex movements are used, and the students are asked to connect the muscles, joints, and movements with concepts from movement science. Examples:

— Washing a window and planes of movement
— Cleaning the shower or tub and center of gravity
— Changing an automobile tire involves a combination of static and dynamic movements

Integration

Link the everyday task with disorders or conditions that might interfere with ability to perform it on a needed basis. Then review treatments or other interventions that might help attenuate limitations or symptoms of a disorder or condition.

— Unloading the dishwasher and degenerative disk disease
— Planting flowers in a garden and hip replacement surgery
— Putting on pants and a vestibular disorder

Diversity Considerations

The concept of everyday activities differs among cultures and socioeconomic groups. The activities and movements selected for this strategy should reflect the general characteristics of the community so that they will be familiar for the students. Gardening, dishwashing, and changing an automobile's tire might not be familiar to all students.

Mime Time 2

This activity involves demonstration of everyday tasks using mimed movements. In this version, all students are given the same everyday task and need to mime the task at the same time. Time the miming for one full minute so that students engage in the activity in a way similar to real life. After the time is up, have the class compare and contrast differences in the ways they moved, how they felt muscles and joints working, and factors that influenced the movements.

Materials and Implementation

Students should wear clothing and footwear that permits movement.

Face-to-Face

Prepared list with a variety of everyday movements.

This activity works well in face-to-face classes. It can be fun to see different interpretations of normal everyday activities.

Online Synchronous

This could be difficult if all students are moving at the same time. Sight lines may be a problem. This could be modified to have students demonstrate in pairs or trios with the rest of the class observing.

Online Asynchronous

Students could prepare short videos of themselves. These could be shared to a discussion forum for other students in the class to analyze

Topic Areas

Anatomy & physiology

Movement science

Learning Stage Adaptation Examples

Review

Observe differences in the movement patterns demonstrated by the class and reflect on how that demonstrates variation in muscle groups involved. Examples:

— Hailing a taxi
— Putting on a cardigan sweater
— Taking a shower

Application

Observe differences in the movement patterns demonstrated by the class and detail variations in activation of different agonist/antagonist muscles. Examples:

— Unpacking a suitcase
— Dusting a bookcase
— Raking leaves

Integration

Observe differences in the movement patterns demonstrated by the class, then discuss diseases or disorders that might contribute to different movement patterns.

— Putting on socks and shoes
— Building a model airplane
— Planting a tree

Diversity Considerations

The concept of everyday activity differs among cultures and socioeconomic groups. The activities and movements selected for this strategy should reflect the general characteristics of the community so that they will be familiar for the students. Hailing a taxi or raking leaves might not be familiar to all students.

Mirror, Mirror 1

Organize students in pairs. They will alternate roles as "Mover" and "Mirror." Students should stand a few feet apart, facing each other, with room to allow movement. Each pair should decide who will move first. The instructor signals the start of the activity. The Mover slowly makes movements that the Mirror must mimic to make it seem that the Mover is looking in a mirror. After a few moments, the instructor says to switch roles, so the student who had been the Mover becomes the Mirror and has to follow the movement. The instructor can have students switch roles several times during this activity.

Materials and Implementation

Students should wear clothing and footwear that permits movement.

Face-to-Face

This activity works well in face-to-face classes. It can be funny, so it is a good stress-reliever.

Online Synchronous

This could work online, but only if one pair of students participates at a time. Sight lines may be a problem. If students demonstrate in pairs or trios, the rest of the class could observe and analyze motor skills.

Online Asynchronous

--

Topic Areas

Anatomy & physiology

Movement science

Learning Stage Adaptation Examples

Review

The instructor asks the class to "freeze" in a position. Then both students hold that position for analysis:

— Joint positions
— Muscle agonist and antagonist activation
— Planes of motion

Application

The instructor asks the class to "freeze" in a position. Then both students hold that position and reflect on how it feels different when they are the mover compared to the mirror.

During the exercise, the mover attempts to challenge differences in balance, base of support, and center of gravity.

Integration

Either when students are instructed to "freeze," or after they participate in a series of movements, they are asked to identify diseases or disorders that might potentially interfere with abilities to perform the same movements.

Diversity Considerations

Some students may feel uncomfortable trying to mimic others—even if it is only movements. If that occurs, recognizing it and working to find solutions will help everyone to participate.

Mirror, Mirror 2

Organize students in pairs. Designate one as the "Mover" and the other the "Mirror." Students should stand a few feet apart, facing each other, with room to allow movement. The instructor gives the Mover group an occupation or sport. At the start of the activity, the Mover slowly demonstrates movements associated with the occupation or activity. The Mirror must mimic these movements to make it seem that the Mover is looking in a mirror. After several minutes, end the activity and have students review their experience as Mover and Mirror. Then the students switch roles and are given a new sport or occupation to demonstrate.

Materials and Implementation
Students should wear clothing and footwear that permits movement.

Face-to-Face

This activity works well in face-to-face classes. It can be funny, so it is a good stress-reliever, especially if unusual sports or occupations are incorporated.

Online Synchronous

This could work online, but only if one pair of students participates at a time. Sight lines may be a problem. If students demonstrate in pairs or trios the rest of the class could observe and analyze motor skills.

Online Asynchronous

--

Topic Areas
Anatomy & physiology
Movement science

Learning Stage Adaptation Examples

Review

Students reflect on joints and muscles involved in producing movements.

Students analyze different planes of motion involved in performance of a sport or tasks related to an occupation.

Application

Students are asked to describe how various positions challenged their balance, altered their base of support, or changed their center of gravity.

Integration

Students are asked to identify how the movements are related to risk of injury associated with the sport or occupation.

If students are unfamiliar with a sport or occupation, have the class suggest questions that could be incorporated into a client interview to help provide more information.

Have the students identify and review quality resources that provide information about the sport, including training, injuries, and recovery.

Diversity Considerations

Some students may feel uncomfortable trying to mimic others—even if it is only movements. If that occurs, recognizing it and working to find solutions will help everyone to participate.

Students may not be familiar with some sports or occupations. If that happens, instruct students to do their best during the activity then take time for class reflection afterwards.

Puppet Master

The students pair up and stand facing each other. One person is the "Master" and the other is the "Puppet." Each Master gives verbal instructions for the Puppet to perform a movement, or sequence of movements. The Master should use movement terminology and is not allowed to demonstrate anything. The Puppet can be scored on ability to execute the exact movements as dictated.

Materials and Implementation

Students should wear clothing and footwear that permits movement.

An exercise mat may be needed.

Face-to-Face

This activity works well as a quick review in lessons on joint actions, muscle origins/insertions/actions.

Online Synchronous

This could work online, but only if one pair of students participates at a time. Sight lines may be a problem. If students demonstrate in pairs or trios the rest of the class could observe and vote on whether the Puppet performed the correct movement.

Online Asynchronous

--

Topic Areas

Anatomy & physiology

Movement science

Assessment and evaluation

Exercise program design

Learning Stage Adaptation Examples
Review

Use a deck of flash cards as students are learning muscle origins, insertions, and actions.

— Incorporate this activity as different areas of the body are introduced to give students a rapid review and build confidence (e.g. direct all movements of the hip joint.)
— At the end of muscle anatomy, have the Master draw several cards and try to direct the Puppet into a complex movement (e.g. flex the cervical spine, abduct the shoulder, and laterally rotate the hip.)

Application

After the puppet has executed a movement—or series of movements, the student pair can review muscles that act to produce the movement, as well as the innervation and blood supply for those muscles.

Integration

Students can brainstorm what disorders or conditions would make it difficult for a person to perform the movement (or series of movements.)

Diversity Considerations

This activity requires students to think on their feet. For slower learners it may be stressful if they have trouble making the connections between instructions and movement execution. Allowing pairs of students to work at their own pace can help everyone get something out of the activity.

Silly Walks

Gait observation is a useful assessment. It can be made more fun and challenging by adding some variety borrowed from *Monty Python's Flying Circus:* "The Ministry of Silly Walks."

Have students take turns as the subject of a gait assessment while performing a silly walk. Students can work in small groups to analyze the gait and describe ways that it deviates from a typical gait.

Materials and Implementation

Students should wear clothing and footwear that permits movement.

Face-to-Face

Students take turns performing a typical gait followed by a silly walk for the rest of the class to analyze.

Online Synchronous

--

Online Asynchronous

Students can be assigned to watch short YouTube clips from the *Monty Python* show and analyze the silly walk gait.

Topic Areas

Anatomy & physiology

Movement science

Learning Stage Adaptation Examples

Review

Describe bilateral joint movements that are used in the silly walk.

Identify agonist muscles acting to produce the movements.

Application

Discuss the role of stabilizer muscles in producing the silly walk movements.

Analyze how center of gravity shifts with the silly walk movements compared to a typical gait.

Integration

Compare biomechanics concepts when the same silly walk is performed at different speeds (e.g. a slower speed involves less momentum which changes muscle activation compared to a faster speed.)

Diversity Considerations

Some students may not be familiar with *Monty Python's Flying Circus* or the humor associated with the program. Context may be helpful.

Some students may feel uncomfortable being the center of attention. If that occurs, recognizing it and working to find solutions will help everyone to participate.

Strong or Flexible

This activity encourages students to explore factors affecting muscle tonus and joint range of motion. A deck of index cards is prepared that lists titles for different occupations or recreational activity (e.g. firefighter, linebacker, golfer) There should be one card for each student in the class. Have students stand in a straight line. Give each student a card from the deck. That is their assigned "role." Then the students must work collaboratively to position themselves in a line organized from strongest to most flexible. After the students agree on their final line, they need to defend the arrangement of their line based upon their understanding of the different roles.

Materials and Implementation

Prepared deck of index cards with enough roles for the entire class.

Face-to-Face

The entire class can participate as a single group or the activity can have several groups of students.

Online Synchronous

Student roles could be virtually assigned. Then the class could use a wiki or a shared document to edit the order of the roles.

Online Asynchronous

This works well using a wiki. But instead of assigning students to individual roles, each student could be required to insert two new roles somewhere on the order of a list.

Topic Areas

Movement science

Exercise program design

Learning Stage Adaptation Examples

Review

Recognize different factors that affect joint range of motion.

Application

Identify activities related to performing the role that can affect posture and range of motion.

Integration

After the class has finished the activity, ask students to describe how active and passive range of motion assessment would potentially differ across the various roles.

Diversity Considerations

This activity requires collaboration and cooperation. Some students may feel uncomfortable voicing opinions that differ from others in the class. Gently encouraging all students to participate can help foster negotiation skills.

Select roles for the activity reflect industries in the surrounding community (e.g. jobs in manufacturing, farming, fishing, finance) to help students make connections.

Observational Activities

Sports Stars 1

Gather photos of athletes in action. Assign different photos to small groups of students. Have them analyze the position of the athlete and identify where the position in the photo occurs in a movement sequence used in the sport. After the students have worked in small groups, have each group present their findings and analysis to the class.

Materials and Implementation

A selection of photos from magazines or websites.

Face-to-Face

This activity works well to facilitate review and give students the opportunity to present to each other.

Online Synchronous

This can work well in an online session by displaying photos online for analysis.

Online Asynchronous

A discussion forum with a thread for each photo that allows students to describe the position. They could also create short videos that display where the photo is in a movement sequence.

Topic Areas

Movement science

Assessment and evaluation

Exercise program design

Learning Stage Adaptation Examples

Review

Describe how the base of support and center of gravity change through the movement sequence.

Application

Relate the position of the athlete to the sport and describe antecedent and subsequent movements related to the position.

Integration

If students are unfamiliar with a sport or occupation, have the class suggest questions that could be incorporated into a client interview to help provide more information.

Have the students identify and review quality resources that provide information about the sport including training, injuries, and recovery and relate that information to the position in the photo.

List tests they could use to assess passive or active insufficiencies associated with the movement in the picture (or the sport in general.)

Diversity Considerations

Students may not be familiar with some sports or occupations. If that happens, instruct students to do their best during the activity then take time for class reflection afterwards.

Sports Stars 2

This activity helps students make connections to repetitive movements used in a single sport. Choose one sport and have students take turns standing in front of the class and demonstrate a movement sequence used in the sport. Have the student perform a few times and then freeze in the middle of the movement sequence. When the student is "frozen" in position, the class can analyze the position. Examples from tennis: serve, forehand, single backhand, double backhand.

After one movement sequence has been analyzed, invite another student to demonstrate a different sports movement sequence. To encourage students to recognize different movement patterns associated with team sports, have them perform different roles. Examples from baseball: pitcher, catcher, or umpire.

Materials and Implementation

Students should wear clothing and footwear that permits movement.

Face-to-Face

This activity can work well in class provided students are familiar with the sport being demonstrated.

Online Synchronous

This could work online with students demonstrating movements on webcam. Sight lines may be a problem.

Online Asynchronous

A discussion forum could prompt students to compare and contrast photos of two different positions from a sport or two different roles.

Topic Areas

Movement science

Exercise program design

Learning Stage Adaptation Examples

Review

Students compare and contrast how the same muscles are used differently in movements for a single sport.

Review base of support and center of gravity associated with the movement and movement sequence.

Application

Have the student who is demonstrating reflect on the muscles used through the whole movement sequence.

Integration

Students are asked to identify how the movements are related to risk of injury associated with the sport or occupation.

Ask the students to find a training or recovery recommendation for the sport, relate it to the movement, and analyze research evidence supporting effectiveness.

Invite students debate the pros and cons of returning to play when recovering from a repetitive injury in the sport.

Diversity Considerations

Some students may feel uncomfortable being the center of attention. If that occurs, recognizing it and working to find solutions will help everyone to participate.

Students may not be familiar with some sports or occupations. If that happens, instruct students to do their best during the activity then take time for class reflection afterwards.

Sports Stars 3

This activity helps students analyze complex movements, kinetic chains, and movement sequences. Find video clips of athletes in motion. Start with one video and watch it with students. Replay the video several times to allow students to document and analyze the movements. Then, use different videos from the same sport or a different sport to give students the opportunity to repeat the activity several times.

Materials and Implementation

Access to a video library.

Face-to-Face

A computer and projector are needed. Students can work individually or in small groups. If small groups are used this can be a team-based learning activity when the groups compare and contrast their findings.

Online Synchronous

This could work online with the whole class or small groups reviewing videos.

Online Asynchronous

A discussion forum with a thread for each video would allow students to work individually or in small groups.

Topic Areas

Anatomy & physiology

Movement science

Assessment and evaluation

Exercise program design

Learning Stage Adaptation Examples

Review

Identify kinetic chains.

Review base of support and center of gravity associated with the movement and movement sequence.

Summarize primary muscle groups that produce movements.

Application

Relate the position of the athlete to the sport and describe antecedent and subsequent movements related to the position.

Integration

If students are unfamiliar with a sport or occupation, have the class suggest questions that could be incorporated into a client interview to help provide more information.

Have the students identify and review quality resources that provide information about the sport including training, injuries, and recovery and relate that information to the position in the photo.

List tests they could use to assess passive or active insufficiencies associated with the movement in the picture, or the sport in general.

Diversity Considerations

This activity presents an opportunity to introduce students to a wide range of sports. Snowboarding, platform diving, and gymnastics are not necessarily the types of sports they will encounter in their practice, but these sports provide excellent opportunities for review and analysis.

Dancers 1

This activity helps students analyze similarities and differences in body position and movement. Look online for photos of different ballet or modern dancers. Find pairs of photos of different dancers performing the same movement. There are variations in pirouette, arabesque, attitude, développé, etc. Students can work individually or in small groups to compare and contrast differences between the dancers.

Materials and Implementation

Photos of dancers are needed for this activity.

Face-to-Face

A computer and projector are needed. Students can work individually or in small groups. If small groups are used this can be a team-based learning activity when the groups defend their findings.

Online Synchronous

This could work if the pictures are shown online and students take turns contributing to the analysis. Small groups could also be used with students preparing a summary and then presenting it to the class.

Online Asynchronous

This may work as an assignment if students are asked to individually analyze different pairs of photos and then post their responses to a discussion forum for the remainder of the class to review.

Topic Areas

Anatomy & physiology

Movement science

Assessment and evaluation

Exercise program design

Learning Stage Adaptation Examples

Review

Analyze joint positions.

Reflect on biomechanics concepts.

Go over muscle group activation and potential variations.

Application

Explore how antecedent and subsequent movements related to the positions might differ.

Identify active and passive insufficiencies that might contribute to inability for dancers to perform the same movement.

Integration

Identify how the movements are related to risk of injury associated with the form of dance demonstrated.

Design interview questions for dancers to gather information to design a treatment.

Diversity Considerations

Ballet works well for this activity because there is consistency to the position terminology and choreography. Students may not have a background in dance, so all of them may not be familiar with ballet. Scaffolding the activity can provide an introduction. Review terminology for the body position, introduce a dance position, and then review photographs of different dancers in the same position. To recognize diversity in dance, look for photos of other dance forms. Have students learn the associated terminology and then review body positions.

Dancers 2

Comparing different styles of dance can help students gain insight into the varying demands placed on a dancer's body. Look for short video clips of different dance styles. Play one video clip a few times for students to analyze. Then, play another video clip from a different dance style. After the students have analyzed both video clips, invite them to compare and contrast how different dancers use their bodies.

Materials and Implementation

Access to a video library.

Face-to-Face

A computer and projector are needed. Students can work individually or in small groups to conduct their analysis and then discuss their findings.

Online Synchronous

This could work using small groups and different videos for each group. Students would work in breakout rooms to conduct their analysis. Then their videos could be played for the class and they can present their findings.

Online Asynchronous

This could work as an assignment that required students to individually respond to the videos.

A discussion forum could also be used to ask students to post individual observations that are different from others already posted by other students.

Topic Areas

Movement science

Assessment and evaluation

Exercise program design

Learning Stage Adaptation Examples

Review

Analyze variations in joint positions and muscle activation.

Contrast differences in muscle groups involved in the different dance forms.

Application

Review biomechanics concepts relative to the different choreography.

Integration

Identify how injury patterns would likely be different in the two dance styles.

Design interview questions that could be used to gather information from dancers about their participation in different dance styles and how that might contribute to injury risk.

Diversity Considerations

Because this activity involves different dance styles, it offers the opportunity to include dance from different cultures. Students could contribute to the assignment by finding video clips that can be used in class.

Musicians 1

Playing a musical instrument involves repetitive movements. This activity helps students recognize how musicians use joints and muscle groups. It also provides an opportunity to review risks associated with—and treatment options for—repetitive stress injuries.

Find short video clips of musicians playing and have students analyze posture and movements. The clips can be of a single musician, or two different musicians to compare variations in posture and movements. Students can review the videos several times to give adequate time to document the movements for analysis. Then then their videos could be played for the class and they can present their findings.

Materials and Implementation

Access to a video library is needed.

Face-to-Face

A computer and projector are needed. Students can work individually or in small groups to conduct their analysis and then discuss their findings.

Online Synchronous

Students can work individually or in small groups in breakout rooms to conduct their analyses.

Online Asynchronous

This could work as an assignment that required students to individually respond to the videos.

A discussion forum could also be used to ask students to post individual observations that are different from posts by other students.

Topic Areas

Assessment and evaluation

Exercise program design

Learning Stage Adaptation Examples

Review

Identify muscles used in producing movements and review innervation pathways.

Application

List risk factors associated with repetitive stress injuries and relate those risks to the movement patterns seen in the videos.

Integration

Identify factors that might contribute to different injury patterns among different individuals playing the same musical instrument

Design interview questions that could be used to gather information from musicians about instrument and how that might contribute to injury risk.

Have the students identify and review quality resources that provide information about musculoskeletal problems associated with the instrument and how they are treated.

Diversity Considerations

This activity offers a chance to look at musical instruments that might be played by clients in the community and also at instruments from different cultures.

The types of movements used to play different musical instruments and practice routines are associated with injury risk. Movements of the fingers for woodwinds, arm movements when playing percussion, and the unilateral motor skills used for string instruments contribute to a variety of different injury risks.

Musicians 2

This activity helps students recognize how music making involves repetitive movements that are different for various instruments. Find short video clips of musicians playing different instruments in a group (e.g. popular bands, orchestras, concerts or marching bands.) View the videos with the students several times asking them to focus on different players each time. Then compare and contrast similarities and differences they observe.

Materials and Implementation

Access to a video library.

Face-to-Face

A computer and projector are needed. Students can work individually or in small groups to conduct their analysis and then discuss their findings.

Online Synchronous

Students can work individually or in small groups in breakout rooms to conduct their analyses. Then then their videos could be played for the class and they can present their findings.

Online Asynchronous

This could work as an assignment that required students to individually respond to the videos.

A discussion forum could also be used to ask students to post individual observations that are different from others already posted by other students.

Topic Areas

Assessment and evaluation

Exercise program design

Learning Stage Adaptation Examples

Review

Compare and contrast different joint movements and muscles.

Application

Identify different risk factors related to the movement patterns observed.

Integration

Design interview questions that could be used to gather information from musicians about their instrument and how that might contribute to injury risk.

Have the students identify and review quality resources that provide information about musculoskeletal problems associated with different instruments and how they are treated.

Diversity Considerations

This activity offers a chance to look at musical instruments that might be played by clients in the community and also at instruments from different cultures.

The types of movements used to play different musical instruments and practice routines are associated with injury risk. Movements of the fingers for woodwinds, arm movements when playing percussion, and the unilateral motor skills used for string instruments contribute to a variety of different injury risks.

Famous Statues

Statues provide excellent opportunities to study the human form, joint position, muscular definition and posture, They can be helpful in movement science to have students understand different ways base of support and center of gravity affect posture and balance. Viewing statues from different countries and cultures can be a fun and interesting learning experience.

Find a collection of photographs of famous—or not so famous—statues. Assign different photos to small groups of students. Have them analyze the posture working from head-to-toe or toe-to-head. After the students have worked in small groups, have each group present their findings and analysis to the class.

Materials and Implementation

Access to a search engine to find pictures of statues is needed.

Face-to-Face

This activity works well in a face-to-face setting.

Online Synchronous

This could work using breakout rooms followed by the presentation of findings to the class.

Online Asynchronous

This might work adapted as an individual assignment. Each student could be assigned a photo for analysis. The findings could be posted in a discussion forum for other students and the instructor to ask follow-up questions.

Topic Areas

Movement science

Exercise program design

Learning Stage Adaptation Examples

Review

Review joint positions and associated muscle activity.

Identify position of joints in relation to movement planes.

Application

Compare difference between active insufficiency and passive insufficiency needed to achieve joint range of motion.

Review biomechanics concepts relative to the position (e.g. base of support, center of gravity.)

Integration

--

Diversity Considerations

In some cultures, statues are used to display nationalist or spiritual ideal. Care should be taken in facilitating the discussion to honor that for all cultures.

This activity could present an opportunity to discuss how statues are crafted to convey different emotions and characteristics of the subject.

Fashion Models 1

Gather some magazines or catalogues with pictures of people modeling clothing or accessories. Students use the photo of the model to review and analyze the position of the body.

This can be done as a speed activity requiring students to list as many joint positions as they can in one minute. This is a nice activity to help students develop a systematic approach to analyzing posture.

This activity can be used as a low-stakes assessment.

Materials and Implementation

A selection of magazines or catalogues.

Face-to-Face

A selection of different photos can be used and passed around to the class. All students write an analysis of each photo. Afterwards, the students can compare different answers.

Online Synchronous

A series of photos can be used and shown to the whole class at once so each student can write an analysis. Afterward the class can compare and contrast different answers.

Online Asynchronous

Students can be assigned photos to analyze and submit individual answer sheets.

Topic Areas

Anatomy & physiology

Movement science

Assessment and evaluation

Exercise program design

Learning Stage Adaptation Examples

Review

Identify position of joints in relation to movement planes.

Describe positions of as many joints as they can within the time frame. Repetition of this activity can be used to help them create a systematic approach to postural analysis.

After identifying the position of a joint, students identify agonist muscles that used to execute that movement.

Application

Review biomechanics concepts relative to the position (e.g. base of support, center of gravity.)

Integration

List active or passive insufficiencies that might make it difficult for someone else to assume the same position.

Discuss how to incorporate postural assessment into intake for a new client.

Diversity Considerations

Among cultural groups that value modesty, pictures of scantily clad individuals may be offensive. To help all students feel comfortable, the magazines or catalogues used should have pictures of models that are clothed (i.e. not shirtless, wearing lingerie, or a bathing suit.)

Fashion Models 2

Gather some magazines or catalogues with pictures of people modeling clothing or accessories. Have students pair up. One student ("Instructor") randomly selects a page with a picture of a model. Then the Instructor guides the "Model" to assume the same position as the picture by detailing the position of each joint from head-to-toe—or toe-to-head.

Once the Model has assumed the position, he or she gets to view the picture to assess whether or not they've succeeded.

For an added challenge, the Instructor student is not allowed to make any corrections. If/when the Model does not assume the right position (e.g. medially rotates hip instead of performing lateral rotation) the Instructor moves on to focus on other joints. This can be very funny when the Model finally gets to see the picture.

Materials and Implementation

A selection of magazines or catalogues.

Face-to-Face

This activity works well to help students become familiar with describing and listening to anatomical terminology.

Online Synchronous

This could be difficult if all students were moving at the same time. Sight lines may be a problem. This could be modified to have students demonstrate in pairs or trios with the rest of the class observing.

Online Asynchronous

--

Topic Areas

Anatomy & physiology

Movement science

Learning Stage Adaptation Examples

Review

Practice describing joint positions, trying to execute them, and getting a picture to help them identify whether or not they were successful.

Application

After the Model has achieved the same position in the picture, he or she outlines the muscles or muscle groups that produce the joint movements.

Integration

--

Diversity Considerations

Among cultural groups that value modesty, pictures of scantily-clad individuals may be offensive. To help all students feel comfortable, the magazines or catalogues used should have pictures of models that are clothed (i.e. not shirtless, wearing lingerie, or a bathing suit.)

This activity requires students to think on their feet. For slower learners, it may be stressful if they have trouble making the connections between instructions and movement execution. Allowing pairs of students to work at their own pace can help everyone get something out of the activity.

What am I?

Study of diseases and disorders can be very dry. But a basic understanding is important for client assessment. This activity turns assessment around. Instead of trying to relate a disease or disorder to a person, the students need to discern characteristics of a disease or disorder. The instructor prepares narratives: a few sentences written in first person that describes a disease or disorder through various clues. The narratives are read aloud, and students write down what is being described. This can be followed by a class discussion to review answers. This activity helps promote listening skills. It also works well as a low-stakes assessment.

Materials and Implementation

A previously prepared series of cases sheets for students.

Face-to-Face

The narratives can be read aloud. After all are read and answered the class can discuss their answers and provide rationale.

Online Synchronous

This could work with a modification to ensure academic integrity if this activity is used as an assessment. Students would need to submit their answers before any discussion took place.

Online Asynchronous

This could be formatted as a quiz using recorded audio readings of the narratives.

Topic Areas

Assessment and evaluation

Learning Stage Adaptation Examples

Review

Students work through ways to identify relevant information and keywords (underlined below in the example for ankle sprain.)

— "I am a common injury in sports that involve running and jumping. Tripping or stumbling can overextend the joint. This stimulates intrafusal muscle fibers (muscle spindles) to suddenly and forcefully contract."

Application

--

Integration

Linking the narrative to anticipated outcomes from exercise helps to identify client-centered outcomes. An example for type 2 diabetes:

— "I am a metabolic disease. Chronic hyperglycemia caused by insulin resistance can lead to neuropathy, blindness, or renal disease. I can be managed with a combination of diet, exercise, and blood glucose monitoring."

Diversity Considerations

English-language learners and students who receive testing accommodations may have difficulty. The narratives should be read slowly and clearly. If this activity is used for an assessment, remediation may be warranted to ensure that all students have adequate learning opportunity.

Dolly and Me

For students who struggle with anatomy and physiology, this offers a creative way to review and can help retain information. For this activity, students are asked to bring a doll or stuffed animal to class. It should be human-shaped (head, torso, arms, legs) and large enough to identify different areas of the body with some specificity. As the instructor describes anatomical structures (e.g. muscles, nerves, blood vessels, or organs) the students palpate on their doll or stuffed animal to demonstrate they know the location.

This activity can be interesting when students work with different types of dolls or stuffed animals. It can be challenging because students will need to approximate where structures are located on dolls or stuffed animals that lack palpable landmarks (e.g. a teddy bear does not have a scapula so the student would need to approximate its location.) This requires more scrutiny by the students.

Materials and Implementation

A human-shaped doll or stuffed animal for the instructor and every student.

Face-to-Face

This activity works well for a face-to-face class. The instructor can easily see when students have made accurate identifications.

Online Synchronous

Webcam required. Students could demonstrate by holding their doll or stuffed animal up to the webcam.

Online Asynchronous

--

Topic Areas

Anatomy & physiology

Assessment and evaluation

Learning Stage Adaptation Examples

Review

Trace origins and insertions of muscles

Identify bony landmarks

Identify location of major organs

Application

Give students origins and insertions then ask them to identify the muscle.

Start with a landmark (e.g. greater trochanter, ischial tuberosity) and ask students to trace all muscles associated with that landmark.

Integration

Ask students to connect relevant anatomical structures with diseases or disorders and then describe a brief and specific treatment plan (e.g. ankle sprain, thoracic outlet syndrome, rotator cuff injury.)

Diversity Considerations

Some students may not have, or be able to afford to buy, a doll or stuffed animal just for this purpose. To help these students feel included, planning ahead is important. Students may need to find a way to borrow one so they can participate in the activity.

Dolls and stuffed animals have cultural connections and often have deep personal significance. This can provide an interesting topic for discussion. As an icebreaker, students could introduce their doll or stuffed animal to the class.

One-Minute Paper

Start class with a blank piece of paper. For one full minute, students write a narrative. They must keep writing until the minute is up. Students can turn in their papers to give informal feedback to the instructor. The papers an also be used to stimulate class discussion. Students can be asked to summarize the essence of what they wrote. They can form small groups to share what they wrote with each other. Then each group can report back to the class about similarities and differences. This can be especially useful at a stressful time in the course when it can be helpful to know if—and how—students are struggling. The One-Minute-Paper can also be used as a self-reflection by asking students to write about what they have learned.

Materials and Implementation

Blank paper and pen/pencil

Face-to-Face

This activity works well as an icebreaker to promote class discussion.

Online Synchronous

Students can complete a timed writing assignment before the class session and then discuss their writings during an open forum in class.

Online Asynchronous

This can be a timed writing assignment submitted to the instructor for a no-stakes assessment.

Topic Areas

Anatomy & physiology

Movement science

Assessment and evaluation

Ethics

Learning Stage Adaptation Examples

Review

This is an excellent review activity to help students reflect on what they have learned or describe where they are struggling. Potential topics include:

— One concept I understand very well…
— Something I am confused about…
— What we learned in our last class…

Application

This activity can help students recognize how well they are drawing upon foundational material. Potential topics include:

— What information from another course has been most useful in this class?
— What does professionalism mean to me?

Integration

This activity can help students recognize how they are using critical thinking skills. Potential topics include:

— What would I do with a client who has a medical diagnosis I have never heard of before?
— How well do I feel I can incorporate assessments into a session?

Diversity Considerations

This is a good opportunity to hear from students who are reluctant to speak up in class.

If papers will be read aloud in class or shared among the students, let everyone know before the activity begins. Students have a right to privacy and should be informed ahead of time how the information they write will be used and shared (if applicable.)

Collaborative Activities

Daisy Chain

A daisy chain is a string of flowers woven together by their stems that can be worn as a hat or necklace. The concept of threading something together can be used in a learning activity by asking students to connect ideas in a sequence to design a private session. Present a case scenario to the class. Take time for some questions and answers so students can come up with ideas. Start at one side of the classroom with a blank piece of paper. Have that student write how they would start the session. Then the paper is passed to the next student who "continues" the session by writing what exercise they would do next. Then the paper is passed to the next student and so on until either: (a) it reaches the end of the class, or (b) a whole session is designed. Follow up with a class discussion about the session design and how it relates to the case scenario.

Materials and Implementation

A prepared case scenario using narrative or an intake form to provide pre-treatment information. Blank paper and pen/pencil

Face-to-Face

The paper can easily be passed around the class. Keeping students on task and engaged in the activity may be challenging if circulation of the paper stalls.

Online Synchronous

This could be modified to use one "session" at a time with a collaborative document.

Online Asynchronous

This could work in collaborative documents with follow up in a discussion forum.

Topic Areas

Assessment and evaluation

Exercise program design

Learning Stage Adaptation Examples

Review

Structure the case scenario with information that references material in a specific course unit. Examples:

— A client with osteopenia
— An elite runner training for a marathon
— A client with relapsing-remitting multiple sclerosis

Application

Present a more complex case scenario that requires Exercise program design skills. Examples:

— A client with osteopenia and chronic back pain
— A an elite runner who developed hip pain
— A client with relapsing-remitting multiple sclerosis who has a sore neck

Integration

Use a complex case and ask the students to include assessments. Examples:

— A client with osteopenia and chronic back pain with limited trunk rotation
— An elite runner who has radiating pain down the posterior thigh
— A client with relapsing-remitting multiple sclerosis who is having exacerbated symptoms

Diversity Considerations

This activity requires contributions from each student in the class. It is a nice way to balance students who are reluctant to speak up in class with overeager students who can dominate discussions.

If a class includes students who have a clinical background, this activity can highlight different ways they might approach session design.

Minus One, Plus One

This is a collaborative activity to help students see how a treatment can be modified. Prepare sheets of paper prepared with a 3-4 column grid; the number of columns should equal the number of students in the group. The instructor presents a case scenario. Each group begins with every student writing exercises for a private session in the first column, then the papers are passed to another student in the group. The next student replaces one exercise with another by writing a different exercise in the second column. The papers are passed again, and the next student replaces a different exercise from the first column with a new one. After all columns are used, the paper is returned to the originator. Each student in the group will have their original exercise program with modifications suggested by the other students. The students take turns reviewing the substituted information.

Materials and Implementation

A prepared case scenario using narrative.

Sheets of paper prepared with grids.

Face-to-Face

This activity works well to engage students in small groups.

Online Synchronous

This could be done with collaborative documents and breakout rooms.

Online Asynchronous

This could work in collaborative documents with follow up in a discussion forum.

Topic Areas

Exercise program design

Learning Stage Adaptation Examples

Review

Schedule the activity so students can review exercises or apparatus. Example:

— Create a whole session using just the chai
— Design a session with a limited number of props

Application

Schedule this activity after students have completed a specific module or course section. Examples:

— Modifications to consider for a client with orthostatic hypotension
— Different approaches for a client with chronic nonspecific low back pain

Integration

--

Diversity Considerations

This activity requires students to think on their feet. Slower learners may feel stressed if they need more time than others in their group. Encouraging the groups to work collaboratively can help.

This activity requires students to provide rationale for their selection of treatment techniques Students who are reluctant to speak up in class may feel uncomfortable defending their choices to their colleagues. Remind students that session designs are individualized so all ideas should be considered.

Rowing Team

Students arrange themselves like rowing teams by sitting 3 or 4 to a row. In each row, all students except one sit facing the back of the room. The remaining student is the coxswain, and sits facing the front of the room—and their team. To begin, the instructor shows a term or concept to the coxswains. Each coxswain selects a related term or concept and writes it on a sheet of paper and hands it to the next student on their team. That student writes a different related term or concept on a new sheet of paper, and hands it to the student directly behind. This process repeats until reaching the last student. Each student only sees one term/concept in addition to their own as each team builds a terminology sequence. After all students have written a word, each "rowing team" takes turns holding up their list for the class to see. The class can compare and contrast how the terms relate to each other. Repeat this activity several times for different terms/concepts in an instructional unit.

Materials and Implementation

Blank paper, pen or pencil

A prepared list of terms or concepts for review.

Face-to-Face

This activity is designed for a face-to-face classroom with room to arrange students in rows. Students should write large enough for the whole class to see their answer.

Online Synchronous

--

Online Asynchronous

--

Topic Areas

Anatomy & physiology

Learning Stage Adaptation Examples

Review

Start with anatomy terms (e.g. bones, bony landmarks, muscles, nerves, etc.) to encourage students to recognize connections. For example, starting with "femur" could reveal answer sequences like:

— hip, sacrum, lumbar spine, ribcage
— quadriceps, patella, tibial tuberosity, fibula
— long bone, humerus, acromioclavicular joint, scapula

Application

Start with physiology concepts to help students make connections to anatomy. For example, starting with "elasticity" could reveal answer sequences like:

— eccentric contraction, Golgi tendon organ, load, recruitment
— stretch, muscle spindle, reflex, interneuron
— smooth muscle, blood circulation, valve, vein

Integration

--

Diversity Considerations

This type of activity requires collaboration. This may be difficult for students who are used to working independently. Efforts to make the activity fun and engaging can help encourage reluctant students to work together.

Students who struggle to master concepts may benefit from seeing evidence of how other students make connections to material.

Dominos

Dominos is a board game that involves laying numbered pieces end-to-end by matching the numbers on each piece. This vocabulary activity uses a similar concept to help students make connections by linking terms and definitions with each other.

This activity begins with one student selecting and defining a term. The next student must select a related term, describe the relationship, and share the definition of the term. The next student does the same and the activity circulates around so each student in the class contributes a term. As the activity moves across the class the definitions a dominos game because one term must in some way match the next.

The instructor can keep track of each term on a whiteboard or flipchart. After the whole class has made a contribution, they can review the list of collected terms and discuss the connections.

Materials and Implementation

Whiteboard or Flipchart.

A glossary of terms may be helpful to use for reference

Face-to-Face

This works well in a face-to-face class. Students can sit in rows or a circle can help to keep the activity flowing.

Online Synchronous

This could be adapted by having the students work in a collaborative document.

Online Asynchronous

--

Topic Areas

Assessment and evaluation

Ethics

Learning Stage Adaptation Examples

Review

This activity can be used to help students review terms and definitions, but guidance may be needed from the instructor to help students identify ways to make connections with new information. For example: the first student chooses "confidentiality" and the next student chooses "privacy," but the following student struggles to find a related term. The instructor might offer a scenario when confidentiality and privacy are needed to help the student think of a related term such as "interview" or "documentation."

Application

This activity is an excellent reinforcement opportunity by using terms from the current as well as previous course units or modules. For example: the activity could ask the students to contribute terms from general professional ethics or relevant to harassment.

Integration

--

Diversity Considerations

This type of activity can be challenging for students who are reluctant to speak up in class. Encouraging the class to be respectful and listen carefully can help students feel more comfortable.

This may be difficult for slower learners and English-language learners. Asking other students to work as a partner by offering clues or ideas, or having students refer to a glossary to give clues can help everyone participate through a collaborative approach.

Connect the Dots

Mind maps are diagrams that are created to visually organize information. Creating a mind map helps students connect the dots by showing how terms or concepts are connected and interrelated through an arrangement of branches/nodes. This activity starts with a theme that is written in the middle of a blank page. Related terms or concepts are written in the area around the theme with lines (branches/nodes) drawn to connect terms/concepts to the central theme. Additional terms/concepts are added to expand the map into smaller branches that radiate outward from the central theme. Once completed a photo of the map can be shared with the class.

Materials and Implementation

Whiteboard and markers or a mind-mapping app projected from computer or tablet.

Face-to-Face

Students can take turns contributing a term/concept and making a connection to another term/concept on the board.

Online Synchronous

PowerPoint or a mind-mapping app could be used assigning one student to be the recorder, use a screen share with the class, and having the students take turns suggesting terms and connections.

Online Asynchronous

This could work in a collaborative document with students making contributions and corrections.

Topic Areas

Anatomy & physiology

Movement science

Learning Stage Adaptation Examples

Review

This can be helpful for students to recognize different muscles and joint movements. Students can select a joint, place it on the map, connect it to a muscle, and then to other joints.

Application

This is an excellent activity to help students break down muscle actions when the same exercise is performed using different props or on different apparatus. The mind map can be drawn to show how variations and modifications are related to each other.

Integration

--

Diversity Considerations

For students who struggle with study skills, this activity can be helpful to show them a creative way to prepare a study guide on a complex topic.

Strips in Sequence

Memorizing the steps in a process or the order of different things can be challenging. This psychomotor activity can help students remember and retain information by engaging them through activity and collaboration.

Write the steps in a process on strips of paper or index cards. Shuffle the strips and place them face down on a table. Have students collaborate to arrange the strips in the order. Once the students have finished arranging their strips of paper, review and discuss their findings.

Materials and Implementation

Prepared strips of paper or index cards.

Face-to-Face

This activity is designed for a face-to-face classroom that has a large table or counter space for students to work.

Online Synchronous

This could be modified for an online class if students work in break out rooms and a collaborative slide to arrange blocks of prepared text.

Online Asynchronous

--

Topic Areas

Anatomy & physiology

Movement science

Assessment and evaluation

Exercise program design

Learning Stage Adaptation Examples

Review

This is a nice activity to include in anatomy & physiology review. Example topics:

— Order of blood circulation
— Kinetic chain associated with specific movements
— Reflex arc

Application

--

Integration

--

Diversity Considerations

This activity may be easy for students with good memorization abilities and very challenging for students who struggle to memorize material. Encouraging all students to collaborate is important so everyone can get something out of the activity.

Plus or Minus

Assessment is both an art and a science. Recognizing variations in how a client presents can help students develop and hone their assessment skills. This activity can be helpful for students to recognize how well they are mastering material.

Prepare a worksheet with a table that lists some aspect of presentation in the first column and has several blank columns to the right. This list might include things like: pain, shoulder asymmetry, frowning, slouching, or insufficient hip range of motion.

Next, present several exercise client case scenarios to the class. Ask students to write a name for the case at the top of a column and then indicate in that column whether each sign or symptom would likely be present ("+") or absent ("-"). After students have recorded their answers for several scenarios, the class can review to compare, discuss, and defend their answers.

Materials and Implementation

Prepared worksheets. Pen or pencil.

Face-to-Face

This activity works well in a face-to-face class to encourage discussion during a review of a course unit or module.

Online Synchronous

An online version of this activity could be set up to have students submit their completed worksheets prior to any discussion.

Online Asynchronous

The cases could be presented using short recordings and students could submit their answers using a survey.

Topic Areas

Assessment and evaluation

Exercise program design

Learning Stage Adaptation Examples

Review

This type of activity is well suited to a review towards the end of a teacher training course or workshop. Using case scenarios that are closely related to the local population can help students recognize the types of presentations they are likely to see in their teaching. Examples:

— Kyphosis in a community with a lot of older adults
— Chronic back pain in a town with a large manufacturing facility

Application

This type of activity is very helpful to encourage students to recognize characteristics of diseases and disorders associated with different body systems that have similar presentation. Examples:

— Back pain in degenerative disc disease and kidney disorders
— Location for discomfort in groin muscle strain and symptoms of prostate cancer

Integration

--

Diversity Considerations

Struggling students may be reluctant to discuss their answers in class. This activity can be helpful to identify material or topics that require additional study or review.

Eager students might try to dominate the discussion in a way that overwhelms students who have difficulty speaking up. Facilitating the discussion can encourage participation from all students.

Project-Based Activities

Where a Client Might Look

The term "ePatient" refers to consumers that take an active role in their own healthcare. They often seek information from nonclinical resources to answer questions about symptoms and treatments. News reports and blogs about exercise and fitness do not always have accurate information. Sometimes trainers end up having to explain or clarify a news report or blog for a client. This is a health literacy activity that helps students recognize where ePatients might look and how to evaluate the information they find.

Ask students to find three different resources that clients might use to answer a health-related question related to exercise or fitness. Have students summarize what they find and rate the quality of the resources. Students can share their findings with the class and compare results.

Materials and Implementation

Computer, tablet, or smartphone and internet connectivity.

Face-to-Face

This could be completed in class as a brief exercise having students work individually or in small groups using a collaborative document.

Online Synchronous

This activity could be adapted to rotate having a few students do this for different class sessions and then present their findings to the class for discussion.

Online Asynchronous

This activity works well as an assignment in an asynchronous class. Students can post their findings to a forum to compare and contrast in the discussion.

Topic Areas

Exercise program design

Ethics

Learning Stage Adaptation Examples

Review

This activity gives students the opportunity to see different ways fitness activities are addressed by the media, bloggers, and other nonclinical resources.

Application

This activity gives students the opportunity to see how primary resources studying or reporting on are connected to news reports and blogs. When information is incomplete—or potentially misleading—students can learn to critically analyze and prepare a response to help educate a client.

Integration

--

Diversity Considerations

Advocacy organizations for diseases and disorders are often used by ePatients to gather information. May sites share patient and caregiver stories. Sometimes this includes personal experiences with different exercise and fitness activities. Students can learn about these types of resources and may gain insight into perceptions and experiences different patient groups have about exercise.

Simple Questions

Using scientific jargon when talking to clients can make students feel important, but it can be confusing for clients. Simplifying information into a client handout can be helpful to use as a guide. Students can also use this exercise as practice for developing marketing materials or social media content.

This activity starts with the instructor listing 3-4 questions that will be used to prepare a single page handout. The students should use an evidence-based approach to preparing the handout. Example: "What is [condition]? Why does [condition] happen? How can exercise help? Where can I get more information?"

Each handout should be only one page with references listed on a second page. The students can be creative in the format and layout. Upon completion, students present their handout to the class.

Materials and Implementation

Computer or tablet.

Face-to-Face

This could be completed in class as a brief exercise having students work individually or in small groups using a collaborative document.

Online Synchronous

This activity could be adapted having students post their handouts to a forum or a few students present to the class.

Online Asynchronous

This activity works well as an assignment in an asynchronous class. Students can post their findings to a forum to compare and contrast.

Topic Areas

Assessment and evaluation

Exercise program design

Learning Stage Adaptation Examples

Review

--

Application

Students can reference information from anatomy & physiology and Assessment and evaluation and apply it to common clinical conditions.

Integration

Referencing outcomes research can help students recognize the difference between direct effects of exercise participation (e.g. improved range of motion) compared to indirect effects (e.g. improved mood.)

Diversity Considerations

This activity can emphasize health literacy by adding a requirement for the handouts to be written at a reading level for 6th grade or below.

Physical Assessment Protocol

The ability to perform assessments evolves as students practice and gain experience. As they learn, students can have difficulty trying to figure out when to choose physical assessments and how to perform them effectively and efficiently. This activity has students create their own protocol to follow to help them develop a process and gain confidence.

To begin, have students make a list of every physical assessment they have learned including gait observation, posture analysis, as well as active, passive, and resisted joint range of motion. Have them organize their list to follow a sequence that is logical for them. The result is a customized physical assessment tool.

Materials and Implementation

Computer or tablet.

Face-to-Face

Students can work in small groups during class then complete their assessment as a homework assignment.

Online Synchronous

This could be adapted as a homework assignment.

Online Asynchronous

The class can use a wiki or collaborative document to make a master list of every physical assessment they have learned. After they have completed their own assessment as a homework assignment, they can upload to a forum for review and discussion.

Topic Areas

Movement science

Assessment and evaluation

Exercise program design

Learning Stage Adaptation Examples

Review

The initial part of this activity—making a master list of all physical assessments—is a good opportunity for students to reflect what they have learned. This could be incorporated at the end of different course units or modules.

Application

This activity requires students to construct an organized approach to physical assessments. Have students share their assessments in small groups to compare different approaches and get feedback.

Integration

Students can test out their assessment tool during clinical practice and revise as they learn. The final result can be incorporated as part of their portfolio.

Diversity Considerations

This activity requires students to apply concepts and organize their own process in a way that makes sense to them individually. Instructors and other students may follow a different approach; this should be taken into account when students share their assessment tools with others for feedback and/or try to practice the tool they created.

Psychosocial Assessment Tool

Psychosocial outcomes are often used in research to assess effects of treatment. The Profile of Mood States, Functional Assessment of Chronic Illness Therapy, and other assessments used in research provide insight into quality of life, mood, and emotions. These may not be targeted as intentional outcomes of a session, but assessing a client's perceptions and experience can provide insight into the value a client places on treatment.

This activity asks students to create a short survey to assess psychosocial measures. First, the students identify different variables they think are relevant or important. Then they can construct a tool using a numerical ranking or Likert scale. After a draft is completed, the students can present it to the class for feedback.

Materials and Implementation

Computer or tablet.

Sample psychosocial surveys and/or research articles.

Face-to-Face

Students can work in small groups using a collaborative document.

Online Synchronous

Students can work in breakout rooms and use a collaborative document to construct their survey.

Online Asynchronous

Students could work asynchronously in a collaborative document that can be posted to a discussion forum for feedback from the class.

Topic Areas

Assessment and evaluation

Exercise program design

Learning Stage Adaptation Examples

Review

This activity can work well to help students review after a course unit or module on the brain and behavior.

Application

Once the assessments are completed, students could apply different assessments to case studies and compare reliability of the results.

Integration

This activity could ask the students to pair their assessments with examples of physical measurements to recognize the relationship among quality of life domains.

Diversity Considerations

The concept of quality of life can vary among different ethnic and cultural groups. Socioeconomic status also factors into quality of life. Encourage students to think broadly about the surrounding community to identify variables for this assessment.

Study Skills

Create a Study Guide

Teaching students how to effectively use all of the materials in exercise science, kinesiology, and education for personal trainers and fitness instructors can help them become more effective learners. Students often do not recognize how multiple types of resources contribute to learning. Instead of giving students a study guide, have them make their own. Organizing notes from books, lectures, and assignments into a study guide can help students review for a test or a certification examination.

For this activity, students work in small groups to create a study guide. This can be to prepare for an exam, or the students can collaborate on ongoing development of a study guide throughout the course.

Materials and Implementation

Paper and pen/pencil or computer/tablet

Class notes, textbooks, workbooks, and assignments

Face-to-Face

Students can work in small groups using a collaborative document.

Online Synchronous

Students can work in breakout rooms and use a collaborative document to construct their guide.

Online Asynchronous

Students could work asynchronously in a collaborative document. A deadline for completion would be necessary.

Topic Areas

Anatomy & physiology

Movement science

Assessment and evaluation

Exercise program design

Ethics

Learning Stage Adaptation Examples

Review

Students can condense material from a workshop or section of the training program into a glossary or table. The focus is on terms and definitions to help students recognize concepts and relate them to each other.

Application

Students could make concept maps of different exercises and connect them using color-coding or drawings to show how they relate to each other. They could also make concept maps of ways to show how different props can modify exercises or make exercises more challenging.

Integration

--

Diversity Considerations

Students have different levels of academic preparedness. Novice students, slower learners, and students from disadvantaged backgrounds can struggle to keep up in courses. Forming groups with a mix of different types of students can encourage peer learning and make this a valuable activity when students show each other different ways to conceptualize material.

Not Quite Open Book

This activity helps students learn to develop and use a memory aid. When resources are allowed to be used during tests, the process of preparing the resource helps students study. Students work during class in small groups to create their own information resource for an upcoming test. The resource could be written on a single sheet of paper, an index card, or even a plain t-shirt (for the students to wear during the test.)

The class can start with a review led by the instructor. The students identify topics that they need help remembering, or information that requires memorization. Then they design their resource. The students can take the resource home, edit, add material, and practice using it. Prior to the test, the instructor reviews the resources to ensure that they meet criteria set forth in class and academic integrity guidelines.

Materials and Implementation

Blank paper, index cards, or plain white t-shirts, and pens.

Face-to-Face

During a review session, students can make lists of information they want to include and then prepare their individual resources.

Online Synchronous

--

Online Asynchronous

--

Topic Areas

Anatomy & physiology

Assessment and evaluation

Learning Stage Adaptation Examples

Review

Preparation of the resource requires that students review course material. The psychomotor activity can help them remember information.

Application

Because students have a resource during the exam, critical thinking activities can be incorporated in exam questions to help students apply concepts.

Integration

Students may be able to more easily learn to synthesize information when they are able to reference a resource that they worked to create.

Diversity Considerations

For students that lack academic preparedness, this is a good opportunity for a semi-directed study activity. When students work in small groups, pairing high achievers with struggling students can provide a peer-learning opportunity. To hold all students accountable to participate, include a self-assessment asking each student to describe their role and indicate the percent of effort they contributed to the overall group effort.

Wiki Me This

Encouraging students to engage with each other and provide support can be valuable. It may help high achievers develop leadership skills and can provide support to struggling students. This activity is a class collaboration on a shared reference resource in a collaborative document or using the wiki feature in a course management system. The instructor can introduce the activity by posting major topics and important concepts then encouraging students to add their own information. This can grow into an encyclopedia for course material. As students add more material, it becomes a place where students can clarify information for each other. The instructor can review the wiki to identify information that needs to be reviewed in class.

Materials and Implementation
Laptop or tablet and Wi-Fi.

Face-to-Face

This activity could be introduced in class for students to brainstorm information they think should be included.

Online Synchronous

Like the face-to-face setting, the activity can be introduced during a class meeting. Students can be assigned homework to make additions to the wiki.

Online Asynchronous

This activity works well in an asynchronous format because it provides an alternative place for students to communicate with each other.

Topic Areas
Anatomy & physiology
Assessment and evaluation
Ethics

Learning Stage Adaptation Examples

Review

This is an excellent opportunity for students to review workshop or session material and identify important concepts.

Application

Students can provide more substantial information by defining and making associations between different concepts. For example, muscle activation during different exercises or variations in amount of resistance used to perform an exercise.

Integration

Students can use this activity to read and analyze a research article that uses an exercise intervention or apply information from a research article to a case scenario.

Diversity Considerations

High achieving students may be more eager to participate than struggling students. When this is the case, encouraging all students to add material or edit to their own level of comfort or ability can meet students on their level. Alternatively, this activity could require a specific number of contributions from each student. This could encourage students who may be reluctant to otherwise participate in the activity.

Short Videos

This is a peer-tutoring activity that uses a creative approach with students creating and sharing short video tutorials (1-2 minutes long.) These could be animations, mini slide presentations, poetry, or music that explains a course concept. Students can be assigned a topic from a list—to ensure that all topics are adequately covered, and then make the videos as a homework assignment. Then, the videos can be shown during class and followed by a discussion. The creative aspect of this activity can be fun while the results provide a way for the instructor to gauge how well students are retaining and applying course material.

Materials and Implementation

Cellphone camera, webcam, presentation or animation software. Computer and projector to play in class.

Face-to-Face

This activity works well as an introduction to a class session or a reflection at the end of class.

Online Synchronous

Students could view the videos as an assignment before class and then bring feedback to the online meeting for discussion.

Online Asynchronous

Students could view the videos as an assignment and then participate in a discussion forum.

Topic Areas

Anatomy & physiology

Assessment and evaluation

Exercise program design

Ethics

Learning Stage Adaptation Examples

Review

This is a good review activity for introductory material. The instructor can compile a list of topics or concepts that are complex or challenging for students. This can be used to create a "library" of videos that can be retained as a study resource for the remainder of the course. Examples:

— Demonstrate how to perform range of motion tests.
— Trace origins & insertions of muscles and demonstrate actions.

Application

The assignment can take a problem-solving approach by having students answer a complex question. Examples:

— Demonstrate a practice interview for a client with chronic idiopathic pain.
— Role-play different ways to rebook clients for a follow up session.

Integration

This activity can require students to reframe a topic or add additional layers of information. Examples:

— Summarize considerations in exercise program design for a client with type 2 diabetes.
— Demonstrate efficient ways to conduct several different assessments before and after a session.

Diversity Considerations

For students who are creative by nature, this type of activity can be highly engaging. However, students who are not particularly creative may struggle to approach the assignment. They may also have difficulty seeing the relevance of this activity. Encouraging all students to embrace different instructional approaches can help them recognize value in creative activities.

Infographic

Infographics are visual representations of data, complex concepts, or processes. Preparation of the infographic requires background research into the topic, organization of ideas, and planning the project. This activity can be done individually, in pairs, or small groups. Begin by providing several samples of infographics to help students become familiar with the concept. Then, identify a target audience for the project, suggest resource material, and assign (or have students choose) topics. Allow time with this activity for providing informal feedback to the students.

Materials and Implementation

Laptop or tablet with an app that can integrate drawing and text.

Face-to-Face

This can be started as an in-class activity with a brainstorming and planning session. Then it can continue as an assignment with the finished product presented in class.

Online Synchronous

This can be started as an in-class activity using breakout rooms for a brainstorming and planning session. Then it can continue as an assignment, with the finished product posted to a forum for the class to review.

Online Asynchronous

This is effective as a self-paced assignment. The final product can be posted to a forum for the class to review.

Topic Areas

Movement science

Assessment and evaluation

Exercise program design

Ethics

Learning Stage Adaptation Examples

Review

This provides a good review for complex material that requires students to link ideas together. This could be done with the entire class working on the same topic, or dividing topics among the class. Examples:

— Biomechanical differences between walking and running
— Effects of a cerebrovascular accident on the body and how that affects ability to exercise

Application

The students can explore interrelated health and well-being concepts to recognize indirect effects of a single exercise session or series of sessions on general quality of life or activities of daily living.

Integration

This is a nice activity to challenge thinking about evidence-based practice because it requires students to weigh theory with outcomes research.

— Identify assessments that could be used for a client who is in remission from prostate cancer
— Compare how different modifications to an exercise affect muscle activation and joint movement

Diversity Considerations

For students who are creative by nature, this type of activity can be highly engaging. However, students who are not particularly creative may struggle to approach the assignment. Having students work in small groups can help to balance different perceptions and help students to get the most from this activity.

Fix My Class Notes

Learning to take notes is an art. Students who struggle with notes may be hampered by identifying relevant information, organizing material, and effectively utilizing notes to study and plan exercise programs. In this activity, students work in pairs or small groups to review each other's class notes and make suggestions for improvement.

Start by having all students open their book, workbook, or notebooks to the same topic. Then ask them to pass their notes to their partner or another person in their group. Have them compare and contrast the presentation and contents of their notes, and make suggestions for additions, deletions, or reorganization. They can use highlighter or sticky notes to "flag" important concepts.

Materials and Implementation

Whatever materials each student uses to take notes.

Pens, pencils, sticky notes, or highlighters.

Face-to-Face

This activity works well to start an in-class review at the end of a workshop or session. After the working session, students can share new ideas or information with the class.

Online Synchronous

--

Online Asynchronous

Students can collaborate through a discussion forum to compare and contrast scanned PDFs of written or typed notes.

Topic Areas

Anatomy & physiology

Movement science

Assessment and evaluation

Ethics

Learning Stage Adaptation Examples

Review

This is an excellent activity to include early in teacher training when students are still working on study skills. It can also be effective later on after students have completed a portion of the training to help them recognize when they might need to find new ways to study.

Application

This can help students who are struggling with problem solving or relating ideas to each other. Color-coding the notes with sticky notes or highlighters can help identify solutions to connect information.

Integration

Students can explain a topic to their partner or group and then review similarities or differences in how the topic is notated.

Diversity Considerations

Students who struggle with notes may feel overwhelmed, but peer learning can be useful in this context. Care should be taken to make sure that all students are supportive of each other by taking a solutions approach to improve/enhance notes.

Some students may be protective of their notes if notebooks are expensive for them or personalized. Other students may be reluctant to share resources. Having another student write in their notebook may feel invasive. To alleviate anxiousness, allow other students to write in pencil or on a separate sheet of paper.

Mind Your MCQs

Successful test taking requires a combination of knowledge and skills. Practice tests are only one way to help students gain skills and confidence. Learning to write multiple choice questions (MCQs) helps to teach students about question design and format. It can help them learn to recognize important information in the stem, identify distractors, and develop strategies to take a test or certification examination.

For this activity, students work in small groups to write a short set of multiple-choice questions for a course unit or module. They choose the question topics, write the stem/problem, and then list possible answers. Once each group completes a short "test," the groups take turns testing the rest of the class.

Materials and Implementation

Laptop or tablet. Blank paper to record answers.

Face-to-Face

This can be a fun activity that promotes discussion when the question writers are asked to provide rationale for their selection of topics and answer options.

Online Synchronous

Students could work in breakout rooms and then all questions could be compiled for the students to use for a practice test.

Online Asynchronous

Students can prepare a practice test to share with the class for review and discussion in a forum.

Topic Areas

Anatomy & physiology

Assessment and evaluation

Ethics

Learning Stage Adaptation Examples

Review

This is an excellent activity to include on an ongoing basis at the end of a workshop or section of the course. Students can prepare mini "tests" with 5 questions on important information they learned. As the students make progress through a course, they would be creating their own practice test bank.

Application

To add a layer of complexity to this activity, have one student write the stem/problem and then another student prepares the list of response items.

Integration

Encourage the students to progress beyond memory-based questions to require higher level thinking. Example:

— Contraction of the rotator cuff muscles produces which movements? (memory based question)
— The activity of the shoulder joint that occurs when a person reaches up to pull a t-shirt on over their head requires which type of movement involving the rotator cuff muscles (memory plus application question)

Diversity Considerations

Students who have been tutored in test-taking skills may excel at this activity. However, students who lack adequate academic preparedness may struggle. This is a good opportunity to take a thoughtful approach to forming small groups so students can learn from their peers.

Peer Teaching

Fuzzy or Clear

Sometimes students have difficulty admitting when they are struggling to master course material. This activity provides an informal assessment through gamification, review, and peer-learning. Each student prepares a two-sided sheet of paper. On one side they write the word "Fuzzy" on the other the word "Clear." This should be in large letters so that the words can be seen by the entire class.

The instructor starts the activity by presenting a term or concept to the class. It can be read aloud, shown on a slide, or written on a white board. Students are given a few seconds to think about how well they understand the term or concept. Then they hold up the sign to indicate whether they think they have a "clear" understanding or if they are "fuzzy" about the topic. The instructor then calls on a student who is holding the "clear" sign to explain their understanding of the term or concept to the class.

Materials and Implementation
Blank paper, pen/pencil.

Face-to-Face

This is a fun activity for in-person classes. If possible, configure the seating arrangement so students can see each other.

Online Synchronous

This can be adapted by using webcams and the gallery view so all students are visible. Students can hold their sign in front of the webcam.

Online Asynchronous

--

Topic Areas
Anatomy & physiology
Movement science
Ethics

Learning Stage Adaptation Examples

Review

This activity can be a good review towards the end of a workshop or prior to the final test out. Allow adequate time for the instructor to give feedback between terms or concepts. This may be necessary to supplement or correct what the "clear" student explains.

Application

This activity can provide an excellent opportunity for the instructor to assess how well the students can break down complex concepts like resting metabolism, energy expenditure, or issues related to scope of practice. Asking a "clear" student to identify resources that helped them understand the term or concept can be helpful to other students—and the instructor.

Integration

When complex information is used in this activity, encouraging the students to compare, contrast, and provide examples can help layer ideas for the students to take away.

Diversity Considerations

The combination of gamification and an informal assessment can help draw out struggling students who may not be willing to seek help.

Hearing a peer explain a term or concept can be useful to collaboratively work through difficult aspects. This interdependency can benefit the "clear" and "fuzzy" student.

If there is a group of students who are consistently "clear" rotating among them can be helpful so that different students get a chance to contribute.

I Could Teach That

Students can gain a deeper understanding of material when they practice teaching something. For this activity, students are asked to identify one topic or concept that they know very well—so well that they could teach it. All topics are compiled on a whiteboard or flipchart. Then students can break out into small groups and teach their selected topic/concept to others. To help manage time, small groups can have 3-4 students with each student allotted 5 minutes to teach. At the conclusion of the peer teaching, the whole class can be invited to reflect on what they believe they did well—and what they learned.

Materials and Implementation

Whiteboard or flipchart.

Face-to-Face

This activity can easily be incorporated into a face-to-face class session. It can serve as a review or an icebreaker.

Online Synchronous

This activity can be done using breakout rooms for the small groups.

Online Asynchronous

Students could write short summaries that they share in a discussion forum with a small group. This would permit the opportunity for group members to ask questions and seek clarifications. Then, all of the material can be shared with the class.

Topic Areas

Anatomy & physiology

Movement science

Assessment and evaluation

Exercise program design

Learning Stage Adaptation Examples

Review

Using this activity to help students review material can build confidence when they are able to identify something that they know well. Example: ask students to teach joint actions or synergist muscles during an exercise.

Application

This can be a nice activity at the beginning of an advanced class or workshop by asking students to review foundational material. Example: a workshop on special populations could have students break down what happens during different modifications to an exercise.

Integration

--

Diversity Considerations

Some students may be reluctant to speak up in class. Having them work in small groups or pairs can build confidence and develop presentation skills.

Care should be taken to monitor groups or pairs so that all students are given an opportunity to participate as teachers.

A Little Help Here

Students may feel lonely if they struggle with course material. Sometimes it can be difficult to identify where they get stuck and figure out how to get help. This activity works through that by operating on the assumption that all students need help with something. Students are asked to identify a topic or concept that needs clarification or more explanation. Each student writes the topic on an index card and the cards are handed into the instructor. After shuffling the cards, each student is given a randomly-selected card. They read the new card and identify where they would go to get more information to help them better understand the topic or concept.

Materials and Implementation

Blank index cards, pen/pencil.

Face-to-Face

This activity can be done within small groups. The students write their suggestions on the back of the cards which can be left on a table for students to take as they exit the classroom.

Online Synchronous

This activity can be done using a wiki or collaborative document to identify topics/concepts. Students can work in breakout rooms to discuss and write their suggestions in the collaborative document.

Online Asynchronous

--

Topic Areas

Anatomy & physiology

Movement science

Assessment and evaluation

Exercise program design

Learning Stage Adaptation Examples

Review

This can be a useful activity for the end of a course or workshop to help students identify resources they can use to help study and retain information.

Application

This activity could be helpful at the introduction of an advanced course that requires students to draw upon foundational material. To help students make connections, the instructor could provide a list of topics/concepts that are prerequisite knowledge. Students would be asked to choose from the list.

Integration

Students could be asked to make a diagram of multiple information sources and grade the quality of the information provided. For example, drawing a staircase that places a consumer website at the bottom, then lists trade magazines, textbooks, class notes, peer-reviewed journals in order of importance helps outline resources for information literacy.

Diversity Considerations

The key takeaway from this activity is the focus on identifying resources that can be used for help, not explaining the topic or concept. The topics/concepts identified by the students are anonymously submitted. This helps to add a layer of comfort—no one knows who is associated with a particular topic or concept.

This activity can provide the instructor with an informal assessment to identify material in need of review. It can also be helpful for the instructor to build a reservoir of additional resources that the students recommend—or use—to supplement course material.

What Did I Say? 1

For challenging concepts, peer-to-peer teaching is often very useful. This activity uses paraphrasing to have students teach each other. Working in pairs, the activity begins with one student designated the "Explainer" and their partner the "Learner." The Explainer summarizes a concept and then the Learner paraphrases what they understand from what they heard. It is important that the Learner not repeat verbatim, but paraphrases. The Explainer listens carefully to identify similarities and differences in the Learner's interpretation of the original explanation. If there are notable differences, the Explainer tries again—using different words—and the Learner paraphrases what they understand. Once they are in agreement, the students switch roles.

Materials and Implementation

This activity should be timed to match complexity of the material covered in the course unit or module.

Students should have course workbooks, notes, and other resources to use as references during the activity.

Face-to-Face

This activity works well in a face-to-face class when the room can be reconfigured to provide space for students to work in pairs.

Online Synchronous

This could be modified to have pairs of students demonstrate the activity for the class to observe.

Online Asynchronous

--

Topic Areas

Anatomy & physiology

Assessment and evaluation

Exercise program design

Ethics

Learning Stage Adaptation Examples

Review

This can be a useful activity for the end of a workshop or section of a course to help students work through complicated concepts. Example:

— How changing arm position during exercises affects center of gravity and balance to make an exercise easier or more difficul.t

Application

This is an excellent activity to help students compare and contrast related concepts. Example:

— The actions of different hip muscle groups during squats, lunges, or jumping off of a plyometric box.

Integration

When students struggle with critical thinking, this type of activity can help them identify key concepts and break them down. Examples:

— What different range of motion tests for the shoulder joint and shoulder girdle would reveal about overall shoulder strength

Diversity Considerations

This type of activity may be challenging for slower learners, English-language learners, or students who are reluctant to speak up in class. Encouraging students to use reference material and collaborate can help them work together as a group.

This activity also encourages students to be respectful and listen carefully.

What Did I Say? 2

This activity uses paraphrasing to stimulate discussion and analysis of a topic in peer teaching. Students separate into small groups. Each group designates an "Explainer" and "Respondent." The class is presented with a concept or problem. The Explainer summarizes an answer for the small group. The Respondent paraphrases the summary without correcting the answer. Each small group then discusses the summary and clarifies information until they agree on their answer. The class comes together, and each Respondent presents the group's answer. The class can review differences in the answers. The activity can be repeated for new questions.

Materials and Implementation

A prepared list of concepts or problems for the students to review.

Face-to-Face

This activity works well in a face-to-face class with students sitting in small groups.

Online Synchronous

The small groups could use breakout rooms to review several questions. The groups can rotate the roles of Explainer and Respondent. When the class comes back together their responses can either be presented orally or added to a discussion forum for students and instructor to review.

Online Asynchronous

--

Topic Areas

Anatomy & physiology

Assessment and evaluation

Exercise program design

Ethics

Learning Stage Adaptation Examples

Review

This can be a useful activity for the end of a course unit or module to help students work through complicated concepts. Example:

— Designing a home and studio exercise program for a healthy adult who has not exercised regularly for the past few years

Application

This is an excellent activity to help students compare and contrast what happens in similar exercises. Example:

— Compare movement and muscle activation of the spinal column in a baseball pitch to a tennis serve.

Integration

--

Diversity Considerations

Some students may be reluctant to speak up in class. This activity provides them with an opportunity to make a contribution in a smaller group which may help them be more comfortable.

This activity also encourages students to be respectful and listen carefully.

Explain that to Grandma

The way a professional explains something to a colleague is different from the way they need to explain to a client. Students sometimes use jargon in order to appear intelligent, but this can make it difficult to talk with clients. Breaking down complex clinical information into easily understandable, scientifically accurate language takes practice. This activity uses a combination of peer teaching and role-play to give students a thorough exploration of a concept that they would need to learn how to explain to a client.

Working in pairs, one student explains the same concept twice to their partner. The first time is as if their partner is a colleague. The second time is as if it is to a friend, relative, or client by breaking it down into easy-to-understand language. The explanation must be accurate, but no jargon is allowed. Then, each pair of students summarizes key differences in the approach and then switches roles to explain a different concept.

Materials and Implementation

A prepared list of concepts or problems for the students to review.

Face-to-Face

This activity works well in a face-to-face class when the room can be reconfigured to provide space for students to work in pairs.

Online Synchronous

This could be modified to have pairs of students demonstrate the activity for the class to observe.

Online Asynchronous

Students could make short videos of themselves explaining a concept for a partner to review and give feedback.

Topic Areas

Assessment and evaluation

Exercise program design

Learning Stage Adaptation Examples

Review

This can be a useful activity to help students. Examples:

— Orthostatic hypotension
— Chronic idiopathic back pain

Application

Students can practice explaining complex topics. Examples:

— The impact of exercise on bone density
— Full body exercises compared isolated joint exercises

Integration

--

Diversity Considerations

Recognizing different ways to explain the same information can help students improve communication skills. This is especially important for students who rely on jargon to try to impress others. Students can practice finding their professional voice through different types of conversations.

Games

Name that Term

This activity is based off of the music trivia game show *Name That Tune* where people compete to name a tune in the fewest notes possible. For this activity teams of students test their knowledge of terms by competing with each other to by trying to identify a term in the fewest clues possible.

The class is separated into teams. The instructor states the general category for the first term. Each team confers to decide how many clues they need to identify the term. The team that states the fewest clues is given that number of clues by the instructor. If they are successful in naming the term, they win a point. If they are not successful, the other team gets a chance to name the term. The team with the most points at the end of the game is declared the winner.

Materials and Implementation

A prepared list of terms and at least 4 or 5 clues for each term.

Face-to-Face

This activity works well in a face-to-face class when the room can be reconfigured to provide space for teams of students to sit on opposite sides of the room.

Online Synchronous

This activity could be modified to have two teams, and one representative from each team competing at a time.

Online Asynchronous

--

Topic Areas

Anatomy & physiology

Movement science

Ethics

Learning Stage Adaptation Examples

Review

This activity works nicely as a low-stakes review when students need to be able to recall information. Example:

— The terms could be muscles and the clues would be origins, insertions, actions, innervation, and/or blood supply for the muscles.
— The terms could be the names of exercises and the clues would be muscles or joints that act to produce movements.

Application

--

Integration

--

Diversity Considerations

Students who are reluctant to speak up in class may feel challenged if they are in a group with outspoken students. Teams should be encouraged to collaborate so that all voices are heard, and everyone has a chance to participate.

This may be a challenging activity for English-language learners if they struggle with terms and definitions. If that is the case, after each point the instructor can reveal the term and definition from the glossary used in the course. This can reinforce the information provided in the clues and give all students the opportunity to review.

Zebra or Horse?

The saying "when you hear hoof beats, think horse, not zebra" is a reminder that there are similarities—and differences—between rare and common diseases and disorders. This game presents the opportunity to differentiate the more common signs or symptoms (horses) from rare symptoms or serious conditions (zebras) that warrant special precautions or referral.

The instructor prepares the list of topics for the activity. It can be the names of health related problems, signs, or symptoms that are associated with the client population or surrounding community. The class is separated into several teams. Each team prepares two sheets of paper: one with "Zebra" and the other with "Horse." The instructor reads the topic and teams are given a moment to confer. Then they indicate whether it is rare (by holding up the zebra sign) or common (holding up the horse sign.) The instructor can ask teams to defend their answer.

Materials and Implementation

Blank paper, pen/pencil

A prepared list of diseases or disorders to review.

Face-to-Face

This activity works well in a face-to-face class when the room can be reconfigured to provide space for teams of students to sit on opposite sides of the room.

Online Synchronous

This can be adapted to be an individual activity with students using webcams and the gallery view so all students are visible. Students can hold their sign in front of the webcam.

Online Asynchronous

--

Topic Areas

Exercise program design

Learning Stage Adaptation Examples

Review

--

Application

This type of activity can help students who lack a clinical background become more comfortable identifying precautions and recognizing urgent warning signs. Examples:

— Shoulder pain in a client who plays squash
— Sudden onset of blurred vision
— Chronic idiopathic back pain
— Unexplained muscle weakness
— Headaches accompanied by nausea
— Hip pain for a client starting an exercise program

Integration

--

Diversity Considerations

Students who have a clinical background will have been taught a different approach to gathering and using information. Students who do not have other clinical training will have knowledge about diseases and disorders that is informed by their family and community. This activity could be useful to guide students into using information in a way that best aligns with scope of practice.

Mnemonics

Memorization is not easy for every student. A mnemonic device is a learning technique that can help students organize, retain, and retrieve information by using a pattern. Students can be challenged to come up with a creative and unique mnemonic or acrostic. A Mnemonic is a string of letters to help remember words or a sequence. Examples:

Airway Breathing Circulation (ABCs) to remember the order for helping a patient in cardiopulmonary resuscitation

Supraspinatus, Infraspinatus, Teres minor, Subscapularis (SITS) to remember the muscles of the rotator cuff.

Mnemonics can be created individually or by working in small groups.

Materials and Implementation
Face-to-Face
This activity can take time to complete, it could be started with a team discussion in class and then continue as an assignment to be submitted later to allow students to refine their work.

Online Synchronous
This activity could start by using breakout rooms and a collaborative document during class. Then it can continue as an assignment to be submitted later to allow students to refine.

Online Asynchronous
This works well with students working in a collaborative document.

Topic Areas

Anatomy & physiology

Assessment and evaluation

Exercise program design

Learning Stage Adaptation Examples

Review

This is a good activity to help students with any information . There are many examples of medical mnemonics including cranial nerves and position of the carpal bones.

Application

--

Integration

--

Diversity Considerations

For students that can easily memorize information, it may be difficult to involve them in this type of activity. It may take effort to encourage them to collaborate with their team.

Students that have difficulty with memorization can benefit from learning how to identify patterns.

Tennis 1

This activity is based on a repetition exercise from the Meisner acting technique that is used to teach actors to listen and pay attention to each other. This version helps students become familiar with vocabulary and terms that are related to each other. Pairs of students stand facing each other and toss terms back and forth. One partner opens the activity by saying a term. Their partner repeats the term and they keep repeating the term until one of them thinks of a related term. That partner says the new term, and then they must repeat it until one of them thinks of another related term.

This activity can be timed for 1-2 minutes for each pair of students. Time permitting, they can switch partners and repeat the game. It works well for a warm-up activity at the beginning of a class session, or a wrap-up activity at the end of class.

Materials and Implementation

Face-to-Face

This activity works well in a face-to-face class where there is space for pairs of students to stand facing each other. To keep the activity flowing, students can toss an object to their partner as they say their word.

Online Synchronous

This can be adapted to have one pair of students participate at a time.

Online Asynchronous

--

Topic Areas

Anatomy & physiology

Exercise program design

Learning Stage Adaptation Examples

Review

Students could use this activity to recognize relationships between muscles and joints by limiting vocabulary to muscle attachments or bones.

Application

The activity could be used to help students recognize connections between different exercises. The whole class could be instructed to start out repeating the same exercise and then think of related exercises. After the end of the activity, pairs of students could share the exercises that were included in their version of Tennis 1.

Integration

--

Diversity Considerations

This activity can help students become comfortable saying medical and scientific terminology. It may initially be challenging for English-language learners. Encouraging students to be patient with their partners can foster empathy and help all students improve verbal skills.

Tennis 2

This is a more advanced variation on *Tennis 1* that requires students to relate terms instead of repeating them. Working in pairs, have students stand and face each other. One student tosses out a term, and their partner responds with a related term. Then they go back and forth each adding a related term until they run out of terms. When a student cannot think of a related term, their partner is declared the winner.

To challenge the class, this can be played as a knockout game. Winners from each round can be paired up to play against each other for subsequent rounds. The winner from the final pair can be declared vocabulary champion for the day.

Materials and Implementation

Face-to-Face

This activity works well in a face-to-face class where there is space for pairs of students to stand facing each other. To keep the activity flowing, students can toss an object to their partner as they say their word.

Online Synchronous

This can be adapted two have one pair of students participate at a time.

Online Asynchronous

--

Topic Areas

Anatomy & physiology

Movement science

Learning Stage Adaptation Examples

Review

This is an excellent vocabulary-building activity to review anatomy terminology or topics in movement science. Example of a sequence of words that can be described as related to each other

— Rectus abdominus: Flexion
— Biceps brachii: Supination
— Elbow: Olecranon process
— Triceps brachii: Extension

Application

One student could be assigned to say only the names of exercises, the other student would respond with a muscle that is an agonist in a movement in the exercise. The next exercise named would need to use the muscle as an agonist. Example of a sequence:

— Pull up: Biceps brachii
— Lunge: Gluteus maximus
— Bridge: Hamstring muscle group

Integration

--

Diversity Considerations

This activity can help students become comfortable saying medical and scientific terminology. It may initially be challenging for English-language learners. Encouraging students to be patient with their partners can foster empathy.

Hangman

This is a low-tech way to review vocabulary and spelling. Using blank paper, a whiteboard, or a flipchart, a student draws out a series of blanks that correspond to the number of letters in a vocabulary word. The other students take turns guessing letters. When the guess is correct, the letter is inserted into the word. When a guess is wrong, portions of a stick figure are drawn to tally the number of wrong guesses. The goal is to guess the word before the entire stick figure is completed. If the stick figure is completed before the word is guessed, the person drawing gets a point. If a student guesses the word correctly, they win a point.

Small groups of students can play several rounds of this game taking turns testing each other on vocabulary. At the end of the games, the student with the most points wins.

Materials and Implementation

Blank paper, whiteboard, or a flipchart; pen, pencil, or markers.

Face-to-Face

This activity works nicely in class with space to configure students in small groups.

Online Synchronous

This can be played using breakout rooms and a drawing software program.

Online Asynchronous

--

Topic Areas

Anatomy & physiology

Movement science

Exercise program design

Learning Stage Adaptation Examples

Review

This is an excellent vocabulary building exercise for any learning content. Example words that could be used from different topic areas:

— Anatomy & physiology: joints, joint actions, muscle names
— Movement science: terms like synergist, antagonist, insufficient, flexibility, balance
— Exercise program design: names of exercises

Application

--

Integration

--

Diversity Considerations

This game can be controversial because it is perceived by some as offensive. A variation is to tally the wrong answers by using hash marks or drawing something different (e.g. tree, house, cat, or horse, or just a stick figure wearing a hat.) A key to the variation is to make sure that there is a way for the students who are guessing to know how many guesses they have remaining to try to figure out the word.

Match Game

This low-tech review matches terms or concepts to help students review vocabulary. Using index cards that are all the same color, write terms or concepts on pairs of cards. Lay the cards face down on a large table. This can work with 9 terms or concepts (18 cards total, 6 per row) or 15 terms or concepts (30 cards total, 10 per row.)

Have students take turns flipping over cards two at a time—to look for a match. If the cards do not match, the students turn those cards face down in the same position. When a match is revealed, that pair of cards is left facing up or removed from the game. Students take turns and keep playing until all matching pairs are found.

For an added challenge, have students create the games. They can work in small groups to create games for other groups to play.

Materials and Implementation
Face-to-Face

This works well for small classes or small groups of students in larger classes.

Online Synchronous

One or more match games could be made using an app.

Online Asynchronous

--

Topic Areas

Anatomy & physiology

Movement science

Learning Stage Adaptation Examples

Review

This is an excellent vocabulary building activity to help students terms from almost any area of the course. This could be played to review anatomy of the lower extremity and then again for the upper extremity.

Application

To help students apply concepts, the pairs of cards can have related concepts. Color coding related cards with different terms could help students make sure that the terms were related. Examples:

— Balance, base of support
— Plane of movement, transverse
— Abduction, deltoid
— Fulcrum, joint
— Extension, latissimus dorsi

Integration

--

Diversity Considerations

For slower learners or English-language learners, this activity can work very well in small groups by providing a low-stakes environment to help with familiarity of terms. Referring to a glossary after conclusion of the game could be helpful for supplemental review.

In a Flash

Students pair up and create a deck of 20 flashcards with terms or concepts they think are most important for the class. One side of the card has the term or name of the concept, the other side has a definition/explanation. After each pair of students makes their deck of flashcards, the deck is passed to a different pair of students to use for a speed review.

One student ("Giver") tests the other ("Receiver") by showing a card. If the Receiver needs help, the Giver can provide clues. The Receiver needs to try to answer all cards in the deck. Wrong answers (or cards the Receiver passes on) are put into a separate pile so the Giver can return back to those and let the Receiver try again. Pairs of students then can swap cards with another pair and play again by switching Giver and Receiver roles.

Materials and Implementation

Blank index cards, pens/pencils.

In lieu of making flash cards a pre-published deck could be used and split up into smaller decks for the class.

Face-to-Face

This activity works nicely in class with space to configure students in pairs.

Online Synchronous

--

Online Asynchronous

Students can use an app to create a deck of flashcards to share with a partner for review.

Topic Areas

Anatomy & physiology

Movement science

Exercise program design

Learning Stage Adaptation Examples

Review

The process of making flashcards provides a review for the students. This is an excellent vocabulary building exercise. It is also helpful for any information that students will need to rapidly recall.

Application

Students get practice explaining concepts and paraphrasing definitions as they build their flashcard deck and when they play the game.

Integration

--

Diversity Considerations

This activity can engage students who are reluctant to speak up in class. For underprepared students who struggle with study skills, this activity can demonstrate a low cost/low-tech way they can create a study resource and use it to review course material. Encouraging high achieving students to partner with struggling students presents an opportunity for peer tutoring.

Got Your Back

This activity is based on a party game that is used to help guests get to know each other. The instructor prepares name tags with terms. There should be enough terms for each student in the class. When students arrive at class, without seeing the information a nametag is placed on each of them: on the back right between the shoulder blades.

The students then walk around to each other and "yes" or "no" questions to try and figure out their term. Once they think they have the answer, they report it to the instructor. When the student has the right term, the instructor peels off the tag and offers it to the student to place on their chest like a typical nametag.

This activity is a good icebreaker.

Materials and Implementation

Prepared adhesive name tags

Face-to-Face

This activity is designed for a face-to-face class where students have space to walk around and talk with each other.

Online Synchronous

--

Online Asynchronous

--

Topic Areas

Anatomy & physiology

Movement science

Ethics

Learning Stage Adaptation Examples

Review

This is an excellent review for any topic. It can be especially helpful for concepts that are not necessarily fun to teach.

Application

Students construct an idea of their term by the series of questions.

Integration

This activity can be helpful at the beginning of an advanced course to help students recall foundational material that will be built upon in that class.

Diversity Considerations

This activity offers a nice opportunity for peer tutoring as students engage with each other and try to think of questions. In cases where students really struggle, the instructor and other students can suggest questions to ask. At the conclusion of the activity, each student can share what information or question was essential to identify the information on their nametag.

Poker

This vocabulary building activity is also based on a party game. Working in two (or more) small groups, students use index cards to create a deck of terms for the other group(s). The deck of terms should equal about 5-8 cards for each student in the class. The terms should all be from the same unit or course module—to help the students with review.

The completed deck—with all cards facing down—is shuffled and passed to another group. Once each group has a new deck, one student deals the deck facedown to all students in that group so they all have the same number of cards.

The instructor says "Go" and each student holds a card up to their forehead. They can see all cards except their own. Students take turns asking yes or no questions from the members of their group to identify their term. When they guess the correct term, they put down their card. Once all students have guessed correctly, each student draws a new card and the game repeats.

Materials and Implementation
Blank index cards, pens/pencils.

Face-to-Face

This activity is designed for a face-to-face class where students have space to walk around and talk with each other.

Online Synchronous

--

Online Asynchronous

--

Topic Areas
Anatomy & physiology
Movement science
Assessment and evaluation

Learning Stage Adaptation Examples

Review

This is an excellent vocabulary-building exercise. Building the deck provides an opportunity to review.

Application

Students construct an idea of their term by looking at other terms in their small group.

Integration

--

Diversity Considerations

This activity offers a nice opportunity for peer tutoring as students engage with each other and try to guess their term. In cases where students really struggle the other students can suggest questions to ask. At the conclusion of the activity, each student can share which terms are easy to remember, and why.

Team-Based Learning

Jigsaw 1

This activity involves small groups using peer teaching, cooperation, and collaboration to explore a complex problem. The activity requires a minimum of three groups and involves three stages.

Stage 1: Each small group of students is designated as "experts" and tasked with investigating a different aspect of the larger problem. Within each group, students work together to acquire information. All participants should prepare notes.

Stage 2: New groups are configured as working groups with students from each Stage 1 group distributed among the new groups. Each student in the reconfigured group has different expertise. As a working group, students share what they learned in Stage 1 to collectively prepare a solution to the larger problem.

Stage 3: Each Stage 2 group presents their solution to the class. Once all solutions are presented, the class can compare and contrast the solutions.

Materials and Implementation

The number of categories of required "expertise" should equal the number of students in each group to ensure all students participate. To use time efficiently, the Stage 1 work could be required as pre-work before the class meeting.

Face-to-Face

This activity works best in a class large enough to have multiple groups.

Online Synchronous

This could work using breakout rooms.

Online Asynchronous

--

Topic Areas

Assessment and evaluation

Exercise program design

Learning Stage Adaptation Examples

Review

--

Application

This is an excellent opportunity for students to organize foundational information into resources to present a case scenario. Examples:

— Hypertension. Stage 1 groups identify risk factors, functional limitations, and precautions. Stage 2 groups would use that information to construct a case scenario to use in teaching.
— Osteoarthritis of the hip. Stage 1 groups identify risk factors, functional limitations, and precautions. Stage 2 groups would use that information to construct a case scenario.

Integration

This activity could be an initial stage to help students utilize information to create a plan for an exercise session or program. Examples:

— Degenerative disc disease. Stage 1 groups could examine risk factors, symptoms, and assessments. Stage 2 groups would use that information to design an exercise session with appropriate precautions.
— Stress management. Stage 1 groups could come up with screening questions for a client interview. Stage 2 groups would outline how they would use answers to the questions to design a comprehensive exercise program.

Diversity Considerations

Students who have difficulty speaking up in class may need encouragement to share within their group. Each student's part is essential. It provides an opportunity to teach cooperation, listening skills, and presentation skills. Depending upon agreement within groups, students may need to negotiate on the solution they will present to the class.

Jigsaw 2

This variation on the jigsaw activity follows a slightly different process through three stages.

Stage 1: Students from home groups and are presented with a large problem. Within each group, they summarize expertise that they need to propose a solution. Then, each student is assigned a role to go seek expertise.

Stage 2: New groups are formed that gather students seeking specific expertise. Each expert group works together to acquire information to inform their particular area of the larger question. All participants should prepare notes.

Stage 3: Students return to their home group and share their expertise. The group outlines a solution to the problem. Each group presents their solution to the class. Once all solutions are presented, the class can compare and contrast the solutions.

Materials and Implementation

To use time efficiently, the Stage 1 work could be required as pre-work before the class meeting.

Face-to-Face

This activity works nicely in class with space to configure students in small groups.

Online Synchronous

This could work using breakout rooms.

Online Asynchronous

This could be modified to have students work in a collaborative document and prepare a video presentation for the final stage.

Topic Areas

Assessment and evaluation

Exercise program design

Learning Stage Adaptation Examples

Review

--

Application

This is an excellent opportunity for students to organize foundational information into resources to present a case scenario. Examples:

— Tension type headaches: Stage 1 groups review the larger problem and summarize what they know about risk factors, symptoms and treatments. Stage 2 groups are formed to examine each of these areas. In Stage 3, students return to their original group, share information, and use the information to construct a case scenario.

Integration

This activity could be an initial stage to help students utilize information to outline an exercise program. Examples:

— Fibromyalgia: Stage 1 groups would review the larger problem and summarize what they know about risk factors, symptoms, assessments, and self-care approaches. Stage 2 groups would examine each of these four areas. In Stage 3 students would return to their original group, share information, and use it to outline an exercise program.

Diversity Considerations

The number of categories of required "expertise" should equal the number of students in each group to ensure all students participate.

Students who have difficulty speaking up in class may need encouragement to share within their group. Each student's part is essential. It provides an opportunity to teach cooperation, listening skills, and presentation skills. Depending upon agreement within groups, students may need to negotiate on the solution they will present to the class.

Debate Club 1

Debating can foster critical thinking, promote cooperation and collaboration, encourage students to listen, and build presentation skills. A debate is a formal argument involving expression of different viewpoints. In order for a debate to be successful, a controversial topic should be selected that has two (or more) sides to an argument. Students can be assigned a perspective to debate. That is especially important when using topics for which most of the class would be in agreement.

For a Fishbowl Debate, two small teams of students debate in front of the class. Each group is assigned a position in relation to the argument and presents their opening statement. Then the remainder of the class can ask questions so each team can clarify or support their position. At the conclusion of the questions and answers, the class votes on the winner of the debate: the team that presented the most persuasive argument.

Materials and Implementation

Students should be given the topic ahead of time to allow preparation. Having course materials and other references on-hand can help students frame their argument and provide evidence to defend their position.

Face-to-Face

This is an engaging activity for a face-to-face class.

Online Synchronous

This can be done online having small groups present to the class.

Online Asynchronous

--

Topic Areas

Exercise program design

Ethics

Learning Stage Adaptation Examples

Review

--

Application

This activity can be helpful when it requires students to analyze and interpret information to frame their argument and support their answer. Examples:

— Pricing affects access to fitness participation in low income or underserved communities.
— Students in group classes should be able to do hands-on adjustments for each other.

Integration

--

Diversity Considerations

Assigning roles in a debate requires students to be objective rather than working from their own beliefs and assumptions. This can be challenging for novice learners. Encouraging students to access information to support their argument can help them more effectively use resource material.

Debate Club 2

Mini debates can engage the whole class in exploration of an issue that has two different sides. The whole class is divided into groups of three. Two group members (debaters) are assigned different sides of the argument; the third group member is the judge. Within their group each student summarizes their position. Then the judge asks questions to allow them to clarify or further support their position. At the conclusion of the small group, each judge secretly writes down the winner of the debate.

The class comes together and the judge from each group reports back to the class to summarize the arguments presented by the debaters. After each judge is finished reporting, all judges reveal who won the debate in their group.

Materials and Implementation

Students should be given the topic ahead of time to allow for preparation. Having course materials and other references on hand can help students frame their argument and provide evidence to defend their position.

Face-to-Face

This is an engaging activity for a face-to-face class.

Online Synchronous

This can be done online using breakout rooms for small groups.

Online Asynchronous

--

Topic Areas

Exercise program design

Ethics

Learning Stage Adaptation Examples

Review

--

Application

This activity can be helpful when it requires students to analyze and interpret information to frame their argument and support their answer. Examples:

— Personal trainers should provide nutritional counseling to clients.
— It is acceptable to incorporate some massage techniques when stretching clients.

Integration

--

Diversity Considerations

Some students may be uncomfortable in a controversial conversation. Take care to ensure that the discussion stays focused on the argument and supporting evidence is provided to support each student's position.

Students who are competitive by nature may be more focused on winning than creating a well-thought-out answer. The instructor can de-emphasize the competitive aspect of the activity by highlighting the key components from each report.

Group work can easily get sidetracked. To keep small groups focused, the instructor can listen in on each group in turn and provide guidance if needed.

Debate Club 3

A Four Corners debate is similar to a caucus. It is a debate on a statement that could be interpreted four different ways: Students form groups based upon their response to a statement. Then each group aims to draw students from other groups to joint them. Each interpretation must be supported by a valid argument. Examples:

— Clients are truthful about their health risks and habits
— Discomfort should be tolerated so clients can progress
— The best way to motivate clients is to push them

Possible responses: always, sometimes, rarely, never are each assigned a corner of the classroom. The instructor reads the statement. Students are given a few moments to decide, then they move to the corner that aligns with their answer. Students in each corner form a team and are given time to work as a group to prepare an argument to defend their answer.

Each group then presents their argument to the whole class. After all arguments are presented, all students have the option to move to another corner to align with a different answer. The corner with the most students wins the debate.

Materials and Implementation

Students can be given possible topics ahead of time to prepare.

Face-to-Face

This is an engaging activity for a face-to-face class.

Online Synchronous

--

Online Asynchronous

This could be adapted to have students respond to a discussion forum to defend their opinion.

Topic Areas

Exercise program design

Ethics

Learning Stage Adaptation Examples

Review

--

Application

This activity can be helpful when it requires students to analyze and interpret information to frame their argument and support their answer.

Integration

--

Diversity Considerations

Strong leaders may be persuasive in gathering other students to their position. The instructor could go around to each group (prior to the presentations) and encourage all group members to align with the argument they feel most capable of defending.

Students may feel swayed to join their friends rather than taking a position in relation to the activity. One way to encourage students to think independently is to ask every student to be prepared to summarize in a single sentence why they chose their location. Calling on a few students may help others feel empowered to move to the group that is more aligned with their answer.

Team Quiz

This activity uses a team-based approach for review and practice tests. It works best with test questions that are complex or tricky. The instructor should prepare a series of multiple-choice quiz questions and answers. The class is separated into small groups. Each group needs four sheets of paper: each with a letter corresponding to a multiple-choice answer (A, B, C, D) written large enough for the whole class to see.

The instructor poses a question with answer choices. The class is given 1-2 minutes to agree upon the best answer. The instructor calls "Time" and a representative from each group holds up the letter corresponding to that group's answer. Before revealing which answer was correct, each group is asked to defend their answer.

Materials and Implementation

A prepared series of questions and answers.

Face-to-Face

This is an engaging activity for a face-to-face class that could be used regularly to help students review for an exam.

Online Synchronous

--

Online Asynchronous

This could be modified to give all questions to small groups, allow students time to collaborate and then submit their answers to the instructor along with a short video defense. Videos can be shared with the entire class and the correct answer revealed.

Topic Areas

Assessment and evaluation

Exercise program design

Ethics

Learning Stage Adaptation Examples

Review

This is an excellent activity to include on an ongoing basis at the end of sections of a course. A session with 3 to 5 questions can be completed in a relatively short amount of time.

Application

This activity can use questions that require students to draw upon foundational concepts to solve more complex problems including client scenarios.

Integration

--

Diversity Considerations

Eager students may overshadow slower learners or quieter students in this type of activity. All students will need time to learn how to effectively participate. Encouraging students to use inclusive approaches will give all opportunities for participation. Strategies like taking turns, speaking first, and polling within the group for the answer can give all students a chance to contribute.

Case-Based Learning

Role-Play

Role-play is spontaneous, contextualized simulation where students take on a persona for a learning activity. The objective can be improving active listening skills, gathering information through interviewing, and/or demonstrating professionalism. Students work in pairs or small groups with one student assigned to the role of "Client" and the other(s) "Trainer." For the role of Client, students are given background information or a scenario. They may also complete a health history form. The Trainer interviews the Client to gather information. This requires the Client to provide accurate responses based upon the scenario.

The activity can assign each Client a different problem from the course unit or module. Alternatively, all Clients could have the same health problem that affects different personas. After the role-play, the Trainers can share what they learned from their Clients.

Materials and Implementation

Face-to-Face

This works well in a face-to-face class with adequate space that can be arranged to allow students to conduct interviews.

Online Synchronous

This could be modified to have pairs of students demonstrating role-play for the class.

Online Asynchronous

--

Topic Areas

Assessment and evaluation

Exercise program design

Learning Stage Adaptation Examples

Review

--

Application

The Trainer could identify assessments that they would perform to gather additional information.

Integration

The Trainer could be required to create an exercise plan and timeline for reassessments.

Diversity Considerations

This type of activity requires students to think spontaneously while providing accurate information. That may be challenging for slower learners. Encouraging all students to be mindful of their partner can promote a quality learning experience.

Students may have difficulty with the concept of a persona. Focusing on the active-listening skills and the essential information can help students recognize the learning potential in this type of activity.

Threaded Case Scenario

A threaded case scenario requires students to follow the same case over a period of time. The basic case scenario is introduced at the beginning of the course then it is revisited at regular intervals for the duration of the course. As students acquire new knowledge, they learn to apply it to the scenario. The entire class can work with a single case or each student can be assigned a different case.

A range of activities can be used for the reviews including having the students write interview questions, identify relevant information, list assessments, or explore treatment options. Students could also be assigned to research information to help them understand the case and how different types of exercise might be helpful.

Materials and Implementation

Face-to-Face

This activity can be a combination of self-directed work and in class discussion with students working in small groups to present cases to each other.

Online Synchronous

This can be modified online to have students taking turns presenting their case to the class during the course unit or module.

Online Asynchronous

This activity could use a combination of independent assignments and prompts in a discussion forum.

Topic Areas

Anatomy & physiology

Movement science

Assessment and evaluation

Exercise program design

Ethics

Learning Stage Adaptation Examples

Review

This activity can be used to help students recognize essential information to extract from a case scenario.

— Case introduction: underline key words or identify essential information.
— Case revisited: identify information from the course that supplements or changes their initial assessment.
— Case conclusion: review again and finalize what they believe is relevant information about the case.

Application

This can be used to help students take a structured approach to assessment of a case.

— Case introduction: identify essential information.
— Case revisited: identify information from the course that provides a deeper level of insight into the case.
— Case conclusion: summarize the case.

Integration

This can be used as a critical thinking exercise where students apply what they learned to solve a problem related to the case.

— Case introduction: identify essential information.
— Case revisited: outline questions aimed at revealing more information to inform their knowledge about the case.
— Case conclusion: review and make a recommendation for the case.

Diversity Considerations

This activity can help students recognize their own progress as they learn new concepts and apply them to a familiar scenario. This is helpful for students who struggle with relevance of course material. Having students work in small groups to present to each other and collectively problem solve can benefit presentation and collaboration skills.

Case Across the Curriculum

A case scenario can be integrated across an entire training program to help students integrate and apply concepts from different areas of the curriculum. This would start with a fictional case scenario that is introduced at the beginning. Then it is revisited in subsequent classes. As students acquire new knowledge, they apply it to the scenario. A single case could be used for the whole class or a few different cases could be used to promote discussion and exchange of ideas. Discussion scenarios can be assigned to different sectors of the class.

A range of activities can be used to review the cases. Students can identify essential information, write interview questions, engage in role-play, list assessments, or explore treatment options. As a capstone project, students could design a complete exercise program including assessments and plan for reassessment to chart progress.

Materials and Implementation

Face-to-Face

This activity can involve discussions at regular intervals.

Online Synchronous

Forums can be used to hold small group discussions.

Online Asynchronous

Discussion forums can be used to have students review cases.

Topic Areas

Anatomy & physiology

Assessment and evaluation

Exercise program design

Learning Stage Adaptation Examples

Review

Introduce the case in anatomy & physiology to help students become familiar with common conditions. Examples:

— 42-year-old male with degenerative disc disease
— 53-year-old female with kyphosis
— 21-year-old male with chronic back pain
— 30-year-old female with asthma

Application

Revisit the case in movement science or when practicing assessments to summarize:

— Risk factors
— Structural and functional changes and abnormalities
— Signs, symptoms
— Possible modifications and precautions

Integration

Revisit the case at the end of the entire course to identify:

— Anticipated outcomes from assessments
— Factors that might influence exercise program alterations

Diversity Considerations

This type of activity can help students contextualize complicated healthcare issues. Including case scenarios that have risk factors related to genetics, sex, and race can provide opportunity to discuss cultural competence in client care.

Requiring students to follow the same case through different areas of the curriculum can provide examples for students who struggle to apply and integrate information.

Creative Case Scenarios

Case-based learning offers rich opportunities in learning through review of material, application of concepts, and integration of ideas. When cases are written or chosen specifically for learning purposes, they sometimes present an ideal or stereotypical scenario. While this may be helpful for novice learners, it does not necessarily serve advanced students. Case-based learning that approximates real world scenarios provides a low-stakes way for students to hone critical thinking skills and integrate concepts from courses throughout the curriculum.

Often, case-based learning requires students to gather information to propose a solution. In a grand rounds format the class works as a single group to review a case. When some students are more vocal than others, the grand rounds format may not stimulate adequate discussion in a way that involves all students in the activity. This is especially challenging when the case seeks a single answer or resolution that can be provided by one student because it limits opportunity for discussion. Having students create case scenarios from an existing resource broadens the opportunity for participation. Creative case scenario assignments can be structured to require either an inductive reasoning approach or deductive reasoning. Both can be helpful to practice observation skills and attention to detail.

Writing multiple cases places a burden on the instructor. This approach offers a solution that provides a learning opportunity for students. Organization using a scaffolding approach is essential for the success of creative case scenarios. This begins with identifying source material, writing and revising the case scenario, presenting the case and using it for learning activities.

Case Selection

Each student should use a unique case to provide variety and also build a library of cases for the course. For a course (or an assignment) the instructor first chooses a category from which the case is selected. Then each student identifies the character, figure, or resource they will use for their case. These should be shared with the class to ensure that there is no duplication of the same case by multiple students.

Using publicly-available information and sources for cases is essential to maintain ethical boundaries. Students can work with information supplied by the source and supplement using course material. As students write their case, they will need to make assumptions based upon the information they can access. This presents the opportunity for students to apply and integrate course material and engage in critical thinking.

Selecting different categories of sources for case material for various assignments or classes eliminates the possibility that a student would try to use the same case in multiple classes. It also minimizes the potential that a student could obtain an assignment completed by a student in a previous class. Although this would not necessarily be expected in exercise science, kinesiology, and education for personal trainers and fitness instructors, integrity is important.

Popular Culture

Writers take great care creating characters that have depth, personalities, individual motives, struggles, and context. Characters also have physical description. For performance, actors are cast based upon physical description of characters. Building case scenarios using characters from books (adult fiction, young adult fiction, and children's books), film, television, or plays provide the opportunity to leverage existing material and build upon it. Examples:

— The television detective Adrian Monk was played with signs characteristic of obsessive-compulsive disorder.
— Walter White (in the television series *Breaking Bad*) had a diagnosis of lung cancer.
— John Stone (from the HBO series *The Night of*) has eczema.
— Eeyore (the donkey in the *Winnie the Pooh* books) exhibits symptoms of clinical depression.
— Red, from Phil Bildner's *Rip and Red* book series has autism spectrum disorder.
— William Shakespeare's Lady Macbeth walked in her sleep.

Biography or History

Biographies and autobiographies provide realistic presentations that can be used for case study. Books often reveal complex details related to risk factors, diagnosis, or treatment including the subject's physical, psychoemotional, environmental, social, or genetic characteristics.

— Lena Dunham's autobiography, *Not That Kind of Girl* describes her struggles with disordered eating.

— In his autobiography, *Lucky Man*, Michael J. Fox, reflects on his struggles with Parkinson's disease.

— Jill Bolte Taylor's *My Stroke of Insight* provides a highly detailed account of the experience of a stroke and the recovery process.

— The film *A Beautiful Mind* is a biography of John Forbes Nash, Jr. who lived with schizophrenia.

— Julius Caesar is reported to have had epilepsy.

— Ludwig van Beethoven slowly lost his hearing, possibly to Paget Disease.

— Abraham Lincoln had physical characteristics associated with Marfan Syndrome.

Bloggers

Coping with a disease or illness can make a person physically, psychologically, and emotionally vulnerable. Some patients elect to share their experiences publicly. Blogs can provide personal, informal insights into an individual's experience with a disease or disorder. Bloggers have different motivations to share their stories. They may find writing to be cathartic, reflective, or a way to express themselves. A blogger may want others to learn from their experience.

It is important to note that blogs should be used only if they are publicly available, written on an open website that does not require membership, login, or password for the reader. Although a blogger using this type of format does not have an expectation of privacy, confidentiality should be maintained when the blog is used to construct a case scenario.

An instructor using a blog as a resource should take into account that information shared in a blog is not verified or fact checked. Blogs are entirely subjective and can provide insight into a patient's experience. Learning to listen to the blogger's perspective can promote empathy. But blogs should not be mistaken for accuracy in terms of scientific or clinical information.

To find blogs, students can do general internet searches for specific diseases or disorders. In order for a blog to be useful in building a case, it should be lengthy (at least 1000 words if a single entry, or have multiple entries posted over a series of time) and have adequate information to get to know the subject. Blogs that primarily post pictures or videos are not a good case upon which to build a scenario if they do not involve the subject providing substantial or ongoing insight into their health and well-being.

The source should be provided for purposes of verification for the assignment, but the name of the blogger and other identifying information should be removed in reporting. No attempts should be made to contact the author of the blog.

Case Writing

Students prepare their case scenario. It can be structured as a narrative, presented as a completed health history form, or other format used elsewhere in the curriculum. The written case can be used as an informal assessment and the cases can then be used for other course activities.

Case-Based Learning

Students can work individually, in pairs, or in small groups. They can present and refine their own case scenarios and use the case for a learning activity. Case scenarios can be passed around to different students or groups in the class to provide opportunities to explore different cases. Potential activities include role-play, identifying relevant assessments, writing interview questions, and/or developing exercise programs. This can all take place to help the students with critical thinking before they start working with practice clients.

Materials and Implementation

Face-to-Face

Cases can be used for informal assessments as individual student presentations or small group activities. Case-based activities can be scheduled at regular intervals to help students practice critical thinking skills. This offers a more engaging approach for students to learn and apply information.

Online Synchronous

This can be adapted for an online class to promote small group discussion. Students can post their cases to a discussion forum for all to review. During live class breakout rooms can be used for small group presentation and discussion. That could be followed by a spokesperson from the small group reporting back to the class with a summary presentation.

Online Asynchronous

Discussion forums can be used to have students present cases to each other and review cases.

Students could prepare video presentations of their cases to the class for review and discussion.

Collaborative documents could be used for small groups of students to draft interview questions or offer ideas on exercise program design.

Topic Areas

Anatomy & physiology

Movement science

Assessment and evaluation

Exercise program design

Ethics

Learning Stage Adaptation Examples

Review

Create cases to help students become familiar with anatomy, assessments, interviewing skills, and scope of practice.

Application

Create cases in movement science to help students apply:

— Known or suspected risk factors associated with a condition
— Assessments to monitor relevant signs and symptoms of a condition

Integration

Revisit the case in towards the end of a course to identify potential modifications and precautions for exercises or program design.

Diversity Considerations

Students have the opportunity to seek subjects for their cases that are of interest to them or have a personal connection. Encouraging students to consider sources relevant to their own community, culture, or personal background can provide an opportunity to inject cultural competence into learning activities that use the cases.

For students who have difficulty speaking up in class the opportunity to work with partners or small groups gives a lower-stakes environment to present and get feedback.

When students have difficulty thinking on their feet, the case discussion may initially be challenging. Allowing the opportunity to revisit the case at different intervals can help students refine ideas and layer course concepts.

Appendix

Appendix A: Sample Lesson Plans

Got Your Back as an Icebreaker

At the beginning of an advanced workshop students will need to draw upon foundation material from a previous course, use *Got Your Back* as an icebreaker and a review.

The instructor can welcome students at the classroom entrance and place the name tags on their backs.

For the first 10-15 minutes of class the students can play the game by asking questions while they find their seats, get settled, and greet each other.

The formal class session can begin even if everyone has not yet finished the game. When there is a break in class, students can continue to work on trying to identify their term. If some student really struggle, the instructor can help with prompts.

Once every student has identified their term and moved their nametag to their chest, the class can review. For the reflection/debriefing, the instructor can share the full list of terms and review with the students how they are going to integrate information from previous training and apply it to new knowledge and skills.

Review with Calisthenics 2

Calisthenics 2 can be used to review the joints, actions, and muscles of the lower extremity.

Prior to class, students should be asked to dress in exercise-friendly clothing and footwear.

To prepare for the class, arrange the classroom with adequate space for movement. When students arrive, store books, bags, and coats off to the side. Have the students sit in a circle or in rows.

Start by having them perform a toe touch. Call their attention to the motion of the vertebral column. Ask them to repeatedly say the movements as they move through the exercise.

Pause.

Then have the students lie supine and have them perform a partial curl up. Ask them again to say the movement of the vertebral column as they move through the exercise.

Pause.

Invite them to share what is similar to—or different about—movement and muscle activation in the two exercises.

For the reflection/debriefing, ask the students to take a few minutes to make a list of the muscles that produce different movements of the vertebral column in both exercises.

Study Skills using A *Little Help Here*

To start a review at the end of course section use *A Little Help Here*.

The instructor can begin class with a brief summary while blank index cards are handed out to the class.

Then students have 2-3 minutes to write one topic on their card that needs further explanation.

Students hand cards back to the instructor, the cards are shuffled and randomly distributed back to students.

The class spends 15 minutes working in small groups to identify resource material (e.g. a specific lecture, book chapter, assigned reading, or internet resource) they would use to answer the question and writes the name of the resource on the back of the card. Then each group reports the questions and suggestions back to the class.

The cards can be handed back to the instructor.

For the reflection/debriefing, the instructor can summarize the most common areas that students identify needing further explanation.

Prior to the end of class, the instructor can place the cards original topic facing up—on a table near the classroom exit. Students can pick up their card as they leave.

Review with Mind Your MCQs

Running a review session prior to a an exam or the end of a course can be helpful. Often this involves the instructor summarizing everything for the class. Instead incorporate *Mind Your MCQs*.

Begin by breaking the class into small groups. Remind them of the resources they were given in the course and the type of material that will be covered on the test.

Then give them 15-20 minutes to write 5 multiple choice test questions.

Bring the class back together and have each group take turns testing the whole class with one of their questions.

For the reflection/debriefing ask the students to share why they identified specific information as important enough to warrant a test question.

At the end of class, ask a spokesperson for each group to type their questions into a shared document or discussion forum to create a practice test for the class.

Appendix B: Sample Assessments

Graded Rubric

A rubric can provide feedback for students based upon expectations for participation in the activity. For collaborative activities like *Rowing Team* or *Strips in Sequence*, create a scale using words for the range of assessment (e.g. Needs Improvement, Adequate, Above Average, Excellent.) Include a numerical rating for each to provide students with a score.

For active learning, possible items for assessment on a rubric include:

— Stayed focused on the activity
— Shared responsibility with group
— Made individual contribution to group success
— Managed time well
— Listened to group members
— Respected other opinions

These topics can help students think about collaboration, communication, and professionalism. Instructors should review and return completed rubrics to students as soon as possible after the activity so the students can reflect on what they did well along with areas for improvement.

Student Self-Assessment

A rubric can be created that gives students the opportunity to self-assess their behavior and participation in the activity. This can be very helpful for games like *In a Flash* and *Poker*. Using a scale with categories can facilitate self-assessment in group activities (e.g. Novice, Contributor, Master, Expert.)

Assigning a number to each category can provide the students with an overall score to monitor their progress. Possible items for behavioral assessment include:

— Met learning objectives
— Took activity seriously
— Time management
— Ability to make opinions known
— Negotiation skills
— Resourcefulness
— Inclusiveness

The instructor can collect these assessments during the course, and at the end of the term, each student can be provided with all of their assessments to review. They can then be asked to summarize areas where they made progress along with areas that still need improvement.

For group activities students can be asked to summarize their major role or contribution. They can also be asked to identify their percent of effort and how that related to the overall effort of the group. Students in a group of 4 would be expected to contribute approximately 25% effort or in a group of 5 contribute near 20% effort.

Grading Materials

Some strategies for active learning involve creation of materials as part of the activity. *Physical Assessment Protocol* and *Psychosocial Assessment Tool* are examples of activities that produce something. Depending upon the program, these types of assignments might be able to count as instructional time. If not they can provide relatively low-stakes way to assess performance and students can also have materials to use in their future work.

Appendix C: Ideas for Reflection or Evaluation

Open-ended questions or scoring sheets can be used for reflections and evaluations of active learning sessions. These can be delivered informally by asking the class for general feedback. Alternatively, brief surveys can be given to students immediately following each session.

Topics for Reflection

— The most important thing learned in the activity
— How the activity was challenging
— What our group did that worked well
— One way this activity helped me grow
— What I would do differently next time to make this a better experience for my group
— My biggest contribution to the group's success

Topics for Evaluation

— Clarity of instructions
— Session organization
— Suggestions for preparation was adequate to help me fully participate
— My time was used effectively
— There was adequate time to complete the activity
— The extent to which the activity was easy or challenging
— Ability to get help or feedback
— Availability of resources needed to complete the activity

Index

About the Author

Virginia S. Cowen, PhD is a researcher, writer, and educator with over 20 years' experience in health, fitness and wellness. She has been a member of the faculty at Rutgers University, the University of Medicine and Dentistry of New Jersey, and Queensborough Community College. Dr. Cowen earned her PhD in curriculum and instruction with a concentration in exercise and wellness from Arizona State University and her M.A. in applied physiology from Columbia University. She is a Google Certified Educator Level 1 and Level 2. She is certified as a strength and conditioning specialist (CSCS) through the National Strength and Conditioning Association and personal trainer from the American Council on Exercise. She is also a nationally certified Pilates teacher (NCPT), and an experienced registered yoga teacher (eRYT) and a licensed massage therapist. Dr. Cowen is passionate about education innovation.

Other Books by Virginia S. Cowen, PhD

101 Cases for Study in Exercise Science and Personal Training
—Pennate Press

Beyond Lectures: Engaging Distance Learning for Exercise Science and Personal Training —Pennate Press

101 Cases for Study in Massage and Bodywork Education
—Pennate Press

Beyond Lectures: Engaging Distance Learning for Massage and Bodywork Education —Pennate Press

Hands Off! 70 Active Learning Strategies for Massage and Bodywork Education
—Pennate Press

101 Cases for Study in Pilates Teacher Training
—Pennate Press

Beyond Lectures: Engaging Distance Learning for Pilates Teacher Training
—Pennate Press

Hands Off! 70 Active Learning Strategies for Pilates Teacher Training
—Pennate Press

101 Cases for Study in Yoga Teacher Training
—Pennate Press

Pathophysiology for Massage Therapists: A Functional Approach
—F.A. Davis

Therapeutic Massage and Bodywork for Autism Spectrum Disorders: A Guide for Parents and Caregivers—Singing Dragon Books

www.ingramcontent.com/pod-product-compliance
Lightning Source LLC
Chambersburg PA
CBHW050711280326
41926CB00088B/2927